THE
CASE FOR
MASKS

THE
CASE FOR
MASKS

THE CASE FOR MASKS

SCIENCE-BASED ADVICE FOR LIVING DURING THE CORONAVIRUS PANDEMIC

DEAN HASHIMOTO, MD

CHIEF MEDICAL OFFICER OVERSEEING THE WORKPLACE HEALTH
AND WELLNESS DIVISION AT MASS GENERAL BRIGHAM

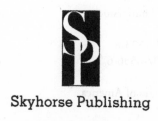

Skyhorse Publishing

10 9 8 7 6 5 4 3 2 1

Library of Congress Cataloging-in-Publication Data is available on file.

Cover design by Daniel Brount
Cover image courtesy of Shutterstock

Print ISBN: 978-1-5107-6523-8
Ebook ISBN: 978-1-5107-6556-6

Printed in the United States of America

Contents

Introduction   *vii*

Chapter 1:   Stopping the Coronavirus Pandemic:
Three Case Studies of Failure and Success   1

Chapter 2:   The Role of Masks in Preventing the
Spread of Infections   12

Chapter 3:   Universal Masking in a Culture of
Community Safety   23

Chapter 4:   Mask Types, Wearing, and Care   31

Chapter 5:   When to Wear a Mask   38

Chapter 6:   Masking in Households and for Children   45

Chapter 7:   Adverse Effects and Discomfort   53

Chapter 8:   Workplace Safety   57

Chapter 9:   The Scientific Basis for Masking: Medical,
Biosafety, and Observational Studies   66

Chapter 10: The Case for Masks: Population-Based
Studies   77

Chapter 11: Developing a Culture of Community
Safety   87

Chapter 12: Masks: The Most Important Public
Health Tool   92

Appendix A: Scientific Research and Medical References 100

Appendix B: Policy and Law References   108

Acknowledgments   *113*

Index   *115*

Introduction

This book explains why masks are the most important public health tool for controlling the coronavirus pandemic. It describes the scientific research that supports universal masking, including observational studies, population-based analysis, and biosafety studies. It provides practical, science-based guidance for living in the pandemic. This guidance will be invaluable in the short and longer term as the coronavirus is likely to persist for more than the short term and may become endemic, similar to influenza epidemics.

I write this book from the perspective of a physician specializing in workplace health in a large health-care system with more than 75,000 employees. After medical school, I sought specialized medical training in Boston including at the Brigham and Women's Hospital and the Harvard School of Public Health. I began my medical career as a staff physician in the Pulmonary and Critical Care Department at the Massachusetts General Hospital and later specialized in care for the health-care workforce at the Mass General Brigham hospital system, where I am the chief medical officer overseeing the Workplace Health and Wellness division. This division provides clinical services for health-care workers, supports injury and illness prevention programs, and conducts research in association with the Harvard Center for Work, Health, and Wellbeing.

I base this book on the experience of serving in clinical and physician executive roles in protecting the health-care workforce during the coronavirus pandemic. Our hospital system's strategy was highly focused on implementing key CDC guidelines. The danger of trying to reduce all potential health risks to zero is the failure to prioritize the safety interventions that will have the most substantial impact. We took the practical approach of emphasizing key CDC recommendations and implementing them extremely well. Our published study in the *Journal of the American Medical Association* describes the unexpected high success of the universal masking of healthcare workers and patients in our hospital system.

Contrary to the beliefs expressed in the popular media and by some medical experts, I do not think we should entirely rely on the development of a silver bullet that will instantly and magically make the coronavirus pandemic disappear. As I explain in the last chapter, we should not expect vaccinations or drug treatments to necessarily immediately halt this pandemic and its continuing danger and risks. Rather, our best available tool to control the pandemic over the next several years may be based on universal masking. We can diminish this pandemic and normalize our activities if we mask appropriately and regularly wash our hands.

While masks are a key public health tool, this book provides practical science-based advice about related helpful behaviors including social distancing, avoiding high-risk environmental situations, flu shots, and self-isolation if you develop symptoms. This practical how-to advice includes guidance about what types of masks are effective, the best way to wear and fit a mask to your face, special precautions that should be taken for children and in households, as well as safety concerns about masking. These are issues familiar to me, as I have answered literally hundreds of emails from concerned employees and patients.

It is important that science provide the primary guidance for how to live and thrive in the coronavirus pandemic.

Scientific knowledge related to the pandemic has developed at a breathtaking rate. Since Chinese researchers published the RNA structure of the coronavirus in January 2020, the scientific knowledge base has expanded rapidly, providing invaluable data for practical application.

Unfortunately, the public has not sufficiently benefited from this scientific and medical knowledge. Instead, they've become overwhelmed by the constant drumbeat of daily reporting by the public media over the internet. Public leaders have provided conflicting information driven by political considerations. This inconsistency in messaging, along with the evolving nature of scientific research and discovery, has confused the public, as has the preponderance of fake scientific news online.

A problem with modern scientific news is that it is impossible for the public to understand the medical or public health context of particular issues. It is difficult to know what science is important and how much scientific evidence is sufficient to provide guidance on how to live in the coronavirus era. This book provides guidance about a strategy for daily living based on scientific data. It not only provides the science behind the guidance for universal masking, but also more specific information about the types of masks and the environmental context for wearing them. It provides a fundamental understanding of the science so that you can make decisions based on your own individual assessment of your risks and medical vulnerability.

Universal mask wearing is necessary to reduce substantial risks of infection within our communities and borne by individuals. We need to create a new culture of community safety that successfully defines individual boundaries, rights, and responsibilities based on shared scientific understandings. We should develop community standards so we can move forward after reopening our communities and establish a new normality in our social relationships and work practices.

   In the first chapter, I describe three striking examples from the pandemic spread that are based on scientific reports of observational studies. Observational studies are fundamental to epidemiological research, particularly in studying the impact of environments on health. In an observational study, the scientific researcher observes individuals to measure associations between exposures in the environment and health outcomes. Such studies may be especially important in studying rare events—such as the current coronavirus pandemic—where collected data can reveal likely associations and their real-world implications.

CHAPTER 1

Stopping the Coronavirus Pandemic: Three Case Studies of Failure and Success

A Choir Practice, March 10, 2020

The Skagit Valley Chorale began its rehearsal by singing "Sing On" with lyrics that describe the changing tides of life that we all experience. The song ends by saying "Find a way to sing, sing on." This choir is known in Washington State for its strikingly vibrant music. Its concerts at the McIntyre Hall in Mount Vernon are frequently sold out. It was March 2020, and the choir was preparing to sing in the Skagit Valley Tulip Festival, which annually attracts more than one million people.[1]

By that time, cases of coronavirus infections had already been reported by public health officials in Seattle, one hour away from Mount Vernon. No cases had yet been identified in Skagit County, however. Businesses and schools were open

---

1   Richard Read. A choir decided to go ahead with rehearsal. Now dozens of members have COVID-19 and two are dead. *Los Angeles Times*, March 29, 2020.

and continued their normal activities. Still, the choir's conductor carefully considered the growing concerns about this foreign virus before deciding to proceed with its scheduled rehearsals at the Mount Vernon Presbyterian Church.

The choir held a practice on March 3. Seventy-eight members of the 122-member choir attended this rehearsal. Four days later, one of the 78 members reported developing cold symptoms without a cough.

Sixty-one members of the choir attended the next practice, on March 10.[2] A greeter at the entrance offered hand sanitizer. They consciously avoided physical contact with each another and brought their own sheet music. Some came early to set up the folding chairs in a large multipurpose room the size of a basketball court. The seating was designed to accommodate about twice the number of members who attended. There were six rows of chairs with twenty per row, which allowed about a foot between the chairs. However, many members sat perhaps 6–10 inches apart from each other.

The rehearsal from 6:30 to 9:30 p.m. consisted of a 40-minute practice for the entire group followed by a 50-minute practice of two smaller groups, which stood and sang around two pianos. Choir members ate cookies and fruit during a 15-minute break at the back of the large room. The rehearsal concluded after a final 45-minute session in the original seating arrangement.

Only one of the 61 choir members had symptoms at the time of the March 10 practice—the person who had developed cold symptoms after the March 3 rehearsal. The member had been ill three days before the practice. Choir members who attended the rehearsal reported that nobody was coughing or looked ill.

2   L Hamner, P. Dubbel, I. Capron, et al. High SARS-CV-2 attack rate following exposure at a choir practice—Skagit County, Washington, March 2020, *MMWR*, May 15, 2020, 69:19, 606–610.

But those infected with coronavirus are most highly infectious 2 days before symptoms and up to 7 days after the onset of symptoms. Shortly after their March 10 rehearsal, other choir members started developing symptoms. The choir director alerted members on March 15 that 6 members had developed symptoms, and those present at the March 10 rehearsal should self-isolate and quarantine. Forty-nine of them developed symptoms by March 15 with cough, fever, muscle aches, headaches, diarrhea, nausea, stomach pain, and loss of smell and taste. Some developed pneumonia and severe respiratory failure. The choir director sent a second email on March 17 reporting that 24 members had symptoms and that one person had tested positive. A delegated member of the choir notified the Skagit County Public Health on that same day, and that agency began contacting and interviewing all members of the choir. Nearly all the choir members who attended the March 10 practice informed the agency that they were self-isolating or quarantining based on the quick communication among the choir members. The individual who was symptomatic before the March 10 rehearsal tested positive for the coronavirus.[3]

In all, 52 of the 61 choir members fell ill after the March 10 practice. Thirty-two tested positive for coronavirus, and an additional 20 had symptoms consistent with a coronavirus infection. Three were hospitalized, and two died two weeks after developing symptoms. The Skagit County Public Health investigation concluded that the singing itself may have contributed through the emission of droplets and aerosols. Exposure increases with forceful singing or speaking loudly in an environment where people are taking deep breaths without masks. The odds of becoming symptomatic were 125 times

---

3   J. Johnson and H. Leibrand. Skagit County Public Health. Summary of Skagit County, Washington Covid-19 Choir Cluster Investigation, 5/12/2020.

higher for choir members who attended the March 10 practice than for those who did not.

The clustering of symptom onsets in connection with the March 10 practice strongly suggests that date as the likely point-source exposure event. The choir members had an intense and long exposure while singing and sitting within inches of one another. No one, of course, wore masks. A member of the choir was quoted by a newspaper report as saying, "It's just normal random people doing things that they love to do, and all of a sudden some people are dead. It's very sobering."[4]

*   *   *

The well-documented and much-publicized story of the Skagit Valley Chorale is an object example of how quickly and aggressively coronavirus infection can spread, even among those taking precautions to avoid it. Specifically, it serves as an example of how freely the virus can spread when masks are not used.

Do masks and social distancing make a difference? The following stories, also involving people working in close contact for extended periods, provide powerful evidence that they do.

Two Hairstylists in Springfield, Missouri, May 12–20, 2020

Missouri's governor reopened the state on May 4, and the first phase of reopening allowed hair salons to provide their much-sought-after services. Few people in Springfield wore

---

4   Supra note 1.

face masks in this conservative corner of the state.[5] The only places in which the city required face masks after the reopening were personal care businesses, such as tattoo parlors and hair salons. Indeed, prior to the public health investigation, the director of the county health department doubted that masking offered protection, saying, "You'd probably have better luck stopping the wind."

Nevertheless, the city's health rules were more rigorous than the state's reopening rules, with stricter occupancy rules in restaurants to enforce social distancing as well as mandatory quarantine orders if citizens became ill or exposed to the virus. The county's health director changed his mind about the value of masking after becoming personally involved in an investigation of two infected hairstylists.

The stylists worked at a Great Clips hair salon in the Plaza Shopping Center at Sunshine Street. A sign at the entrance announced to all customers that "a mask is required." One of the stylists developed a cough and fever on May 12 but continued to work, thinking that the symptoms were due to allergies. She wore a mask while working as required by company policy, except for time spent with another stylist during breaks from work. She continued to work for eight days until she was tested. During that time, she had been exposed to 84 customers for 15 to 45 minutes apiece while cutting their hair and providing other personal care services.

The second stylist was closely exposed to the first during work breaks, when neither were wearing masks. She developed mild respiratory symptoms on May 15 but continued working for five more days before being tested, caring for 56 clients while wearing a mask. The county health department used Great Clip's electronic reservation system to

5 Todd C. Frankel. The outbreak that didn't happen: Masks credited with preventing coronavirus spread inside Missouri hair salon, *Washington Post*, June 17, 2020.

identify the 139 clients who had been closely exposed to the two hairstylists.

The Green County Health Department conducted contact tracing for all 139 of these clients. The department determined that the first stylist always wore a double-layered cotton face covering when with her clients, and the second stylist likewise always wore a double-layered cotton mask or sometimes a surgical mask. Ninety-eight percent of the clients reported wearing a mask, with the remainder not being able to recall.

The 139 clients were quarantined for 14 days. Despite their prolonged close exposure with the infected hairstylists, none of the clients developed symptoms or tested positive for coronavirus. Sixty-seven volunteered to be tested, and all tested negative. The household contacts of the two stylists were also contacted. All four members of the first stylist's household developed symptoms and had positive tests. Fortunately, the two other members of the second stylist's household did not develop symptoms. The published study of the data connected to the public health investigation concluded that the exposed customers were likely protected from infection by the community's and company's masking policies.[6]

The Mass General Brigham Hospital System's Universal Masking of Workers and Patients, March 25, 2020

The Mass General Brigham (known by its acronym, "MGB") is one of the most highly respected hospital systems in the world. It includes two academic medical centers affiliated with the Harvard Medical School, the Massachusetts General

---

6   M. J. Hendrix, C. Walde, K. Findley, and R. Trotman. Absence of apparent transmission of SARS-CoV-2 from two stylists after exposure at a hair salon with a universal face covering policy—Springfield, Missouri, May 2020, *MMWR*, July 17, 2020 69(28):930–932.

Hospital and the Brigham and Women's Hospital. It is the largest hospital system in Massachusetts with more than 78,000 employees and 12 hospitals. Its hospitals have illustrious histories and have pioneered many important advances in medical care. The Mass General Hospital was the first hospital to successfully use general anesthesia for surgery, and the Brigham and Women's Hospital was the first to initiate cardiac valve surgeries.

Less known is the fact that these hospitals have led the way in the study and treatment of environmental and workplace illnesses, a medical specialty founded by Drs. Alice Hamilton and Harriet Hardy at the Massachusetts General Hospital. Given MGB's intellectual heritage, it should be no surprise that the MGB has also led the way in establishing universal masking of workers and patients during the coronavirus pandemic.

At the beginning of the pandemic's spread to Massachusetts in March, the hospital system's leadership made the bold decision to require the masking of all employees and patients in its hospitals. While universal masking is now the norm for hospitals, MGB was likely the first hospital system in the country to make this enormous resource commitment. Large supplies of personal protective equipment were scarce, and tens of thousands of surgical masks had to be provided for regular daily use. In an editorial in the *New England Journal of Medicine*, the MGB hospital infection control and administrative leaders noted that only "a handful" of American hospitals even by late May had adopted a mandatory universal masking policy, although this had become the standard in a number of hospitals in Asia.[7]

---

7   M. Klompas, C. A. Morris, J. Sinclair, M. Pearson, and E. S. Shenoy. Universal masking in hospitals in the Covid-19 era. *New England Journal of Medicine*, May 21, 2020, 382:e63.

The data from MGB's universal masking program is ideal for research study for several reasons. The employee health services established a large service center at the start of the pandemic so that its employees could arrange for testing by phone call if they had symptoms. The primary criterion for testing health-care workers was the presence of symptoms consistent with a coronavirus infection. The number of workers tested daily remained stable from before the onset of the pandemic in Massachusetts to after the imposition of universal masking in March and April, when the daily number of new coronavirus infections in the state was continuing to increase.

Before the adoption of the mandatory masking policy from March 6 to March 25, the positive test rate (a common metric based on the proportion of positive tests of the total tests) among hospital workers was rising exponentially, from 0 percent to 21.32 percent. The rate of positive test results increased by a mean average of 1.16 percent per day, with cases doubling every 3.6 days.

But shortly after March 25, when masking was first required of workers, there appeared to be an abrupt fall in the positive test rate. Rates further decreased following the masking of patients on April 6. After this intervention period, the positive test rate among hospital workers decreased linearly from 14.65 percent to 11.46 percent.[8]

The fall in the positive test rate among hospital workers reached a point where it largely reflected the rate of infection in the communities where they lived. The renowned medical writer and thinker Dr. Atul Gawande discussed the MGB hospital data with the infection control leader of the Brigham and Women's Hospital and concluded there were

8   X. Wang, E. G. Ferro, G. Zhou, D. Hashimoto, and D. L. Bhatt. Association between universal masking in a health care system and SARS-CoV-2 positivity among health care workers. *Journal of the American Medical Association*, July 14, 2020, E1–E2.

"few workplace transmissions." He observed that the MGB hospitals have "learned to avoid becoming sites of spread."[9] Given the vulnerability of hospital workplaces to the coronavirus spread, this was a remarkable and unexpected achievement, and directly due to mandatory masking.

* * *

When the MGB study was published in the *Journal of the American Medical Association* on July 14, 2020, the director of the Centers for Disease Control and Prevention (CDC), Dr. Robert Redfield, and other leaders of his agency published an editorial in the same journal issue. Dr. Redfield has been a national leader in public health for 30 years as well as a world authority in virology research. The CDC editorial described the MGB study as providing "critically important data to emphasize that masking helps prevent transmission" of the coronavirus. It further concluded that the decreases in positive testing rates among the health-care workers in the MGB study were "unlikely to be artifactual" because the number of tested symptomatic workers per day remained consistent even as the daily number of new coronavirus infections in the state continued to increase or plateau.[10]

Dr. Redfield and his colleagues argued that the findings from the MGB study can be generalized to universal public masking, since they show the benefits of masking in situations where people are physically close to each other and social distancing is not possible—health-care workers can rarely socially distance while caring for their patients. They

---

9   Atul Gawande. Amid the coronavirus crisis, a regimen for reentry. *The New Yorker*, May 13, 2020.

10 J. T. Brooks, J. C. Butler, and R. R. Redfield. Universal masking to prevent SARS-CoV-2 transmission—The time is Now, *Journal of the American Medical Association*, July 14, 2020, E1-E2.

compared the potential impact of masking to that of vaccines in creating herd immunity: The more individuals wear cloth coverings, the greater the public protection against the virus.

The CDC editorial also noted online surveys showing the public was adopting cloth face coverings. The self-reported prevalence of mask use when away from home rose from 61.9 percent to 76.4 percent during May 11–13, 2020. Noting the significance of the study of the two infected hairstylists, the CDC leaders also cited a study by Goldman Sachs Research indicating that expanding community masking by 15 percent could save 5 percent of gross domestic product, about $1 trillion, by preventing the need for stay-at-home orders in states with rising infection rates.

The CDC's strong recommendation for universal public masking represents a complete reversal from its initial recommendations at the time the first coronavirus case in the United States was identified on January 30. At that time, the CDC chose not to recommend masks to the public. Unlike Asian countries, which had long experience in public mask-wearing since the 2002 SARS epidemic, the United States had not adopted masking as an acceptable public practice. And while there was already scientific evidence supporting masks, the CDC was concerned about potential public hoarding of medical-grade masks, as had occurred for hand sanitizers and toilet paper. On February 27, Dr. Redfield himself said, "There is no role for these masks in the community. These masks need to be prioritized for health professions that as part of their job are taking care of individuals." The president and vice president notably did not wear masks in public at that time.

But on April 3, the CDC modified its guidance by recommending that the public consider wearing cloth masks that could be made at home, particularly in areas of the country with a high transmission of infection. It pointed to growing scientific evidence indicating masks may help prevent the spreading of the virus when those infected remain asymptomatic and do not develop symptoms or are presymptomatic—that is, infected but not yet showing symptoms.

The CDC's declaration that the time for universal masking is now made it clear there was a sea change in policy. On news broadcasts following the July 14 editorial, Dr. Redfield concluded, "We are not defenseless against this virus. . . . If all of us would put on a face covering in the next 4 to 6 weeks, we can drive this epidemic into the ground."

The CDC director's call to arms represented a turning point in our war on the coronavirus. In the following week, the NIH director appeared on the Sunday-morning television show *Face the Nation* wearing a mask at the start of the interview to emphasize support. Later, the president appeared before the national press wearing a mask, despite having previously and repeatedly expressed his skepticism. A couple weeks later, major health organizations announced their public support for universal masking, including the American Medical Association, the American Hospital Association, and the American Nursing Association.

The changing tide in support of masks was sparked by the striking evidence emerging from the scientifically documented narratives of recent pandemic experiences: Consistent, universal mask wearing works. The next chapters will explore the role of mask-wearing and building a culture that promotes public health and safety.

CHAPTER 2

The Role of Masks in Preventing the Spread of Infections

In this chapter, I will show that universal masking is an effective way to prevent infection when used as part of a four-point strategy that includes washing hands, a daily symptom check, and social distancing. I start this chapter with an overview of the scientific basis for masking and evidence for its effectiveness. Next, I provide practical guidance for the other three pillars of infection prevention—hand-washing, daily symptom checks, and social distancing. If we are diligent in abiding by these safe behaviors, the pandemic could be effectively managed and diminished.

The Central Role of Masks

To understand how to stop viral infections such as COVID-19 from spreading, we must first understand the dynamics of viral spread. Respiratory droplets produced by coughing, talking, or just exhaling are the primary source of infection. These invisible droplets of moisture usually fall within six feet and can land in the mouths or noses of nearby people or be inhaled by them. Forceful coughing can propel respiratory droplets up to 20 feet. Thus, besides wearing a mask, the person about to cough should block it with an elbow or tissue and turn away from others to avoid infecting them.

The most common risk of infection, however, comes from quietly exhaled and invisible droplets that may transmit disease within six feet. Transmission of these droplets can be effectively blocked by masks, and surgical masks may block 95–99 percent of respiratory droplets from being exhaled by the wearer.[1] The double-layered cotton used by many for cloth masking may also be highly effective, blocking about 60 percent of droplets. An international consortium of scientists concluded that if 60 percent of the world's population were to wear masks having this level of effectiveness, the pandemic could be stopped.[2]

In some instances, the respiratory particles may be tinier than droplets and likely to travel further by aerosolizing into finer particulates that persist longer in the air, perhaps hours. There is controversy about how often aerosolization occurs, but the CDC, WHO, and most scientists do not currently believe it to be a common means of infection in public areas. Some experts point out, however, that the aerosolization of the virus, affected perhaps by ventilation, humidity, and other environmental factors, may occur in certain crowded indoor settings such as restaurants or conferences, making a super-spreading event possible among those not wearing masks.[3] In a hospital setting, we require N-95 respirators for hospital workers who work in close proximity to certain

---

1   N. H. Leung, D. K. W. Chu, E. Y. Shieu et al. Respiratory virus shedding in exhaled breath and efficacy of face masks. *Nature Medicine* 26, 676–680 (2020).

2   Howard, J.; Huang, A.; Li, Z.; Tufekci, Z.; et al. Face Masks Against COVID-19: An Evidence Review. *Preprints* 2020, 2020040203 (doi: 10.20944/preprints202004.0203.v1).

3   M. Klompas, M. A. Baker, and C. Rhee. Airborne Transmission of SARS-CoV-2: Theoretical Considerations and Available Evidence. *JAMA.* 2020;324(5):441–442. doi:10.1001/jama.2020.12458

aerosolizing procedures, such as pulmonary specialists performing bronchoscopies on patients.

Even if a person has no symptoms, he or she may still be exposing others to the coronavirus. Indeed, up to 30 to 40 percent of those infected are asymptomatic, yet may be exhaling the same amount of virus as someone who is symptomatic. Moreover, those who become infected are infectious for 1–2 days prior to having symptoms. Thus, a major contributor to infection is the invisible and silent nature of exposure from those infected. For this reason, universal masking in public areas must be the primary way to control the insidious spread of the pandemic.

Based on current science, the main purpose of masking is to prevent the mask wearer from infecting others. It is generally thought that wearing a mask does not provide sufficient protection for the wearer from infection by respiratory droplets, unlike wearing respirators such as N-95s. However, there is limited scientific evidence that points to the possibility that people wearing masks may be protected from infection in some cases. Masks may reduce the inhalation of droplets by 35 to 75 percent depending on the type and fit of the mask. During the SARS outbreak in Hong Kong, people who wore masks frequently in public were half as likely to report being infected as those who did not.[4]

Similarly, there is some evidence that wearing a mask may limit the risk of serious illness by reducing the amount of viral exposure. In situations where mandatory masking was enforced (on a cruise ship, in a seafood-processing plant, and in a meat-processing plant), the proportion of asymptomatic infections was between 81 and 95 percent. It has been hypothesized that the high proportion of asymptomatic infections

4   J. Lau, H. Tsui, M. Lau, et al. SARS Transmission, Risk Factors, and Prevention in Hong Kong. *Emerging Infectious Diseases*. 2004;10(4):587–592. doi:10.3201/eid1004.030628.

may have resulted from the lower dose of viral exposure associated with the universal masking. However, our hospitals show infection data consistent with published data from other hospitals where universal masking is in place: The prevalence of positive antibody tests of those not reporting infection was less than 2 percent among health-care workers.[5] The hospital data thus contradict the hypothesis that universal masking is linked to higher rates of asymptomatic infections.

Within the MGB hospital system, we require that workers and patients use hand sanitizer, then put on surgical masks at the hospital entrance. This prevents the silent spreading of infections by exhaled respiratory droplets within hospital community. As a society, we need to find ways to expand the availability of masks so it becomes customary to put on a face covering when leaving our homes or before opening our car doors and entering into public spaces.

This raises the question of how long one can safely go unmasked in a public area. Or phrased more precisely, what constitutes a significant period of exposure to coronavirus if a mask is not worn or slips out of position over the nose and mouth? The CDC definition of a significant exposure event is one in which an individual (who may be masked) in a hospital setting is within six feet of another person who is not wearing a mask, such as a fellow worker or patient, for 15 minutes. Through exposure tracing, an infection control and occupational team conducts exposure tracing to determine if there are significant exposures to coronavirus and notifies those who may have been exposed. If a person has

---

5   See J. Moscola, G. Sembajwe, M. Jarrett, et al. Prevalence of SARS-CoV-2 antibodies in health care personnel in the New York cit area. *JAMA*. August 6, 2020.; F. S. Vahidy, D. W. Bernard, M. L. Boom, et al. Prevalence of SARS-CoV-2 infection among asymptomatic health care workers in the greater Houston, Texas, Area. *JAMA* NMetw open 2020;3(7): e206451. Doi:10.1001 /jamanetworkopen.2020.16451.

been exposed for 15 or more minutes in such conditions, it is critical that this person conduct careful symptom monitoring for the following 14 days and get testing within 2 to 10 days. In short, it is important to consistently wear a mask in public spaces, especially when social distancing cannot be maintained.

Masking as Part of a Four-Point Strategy of Prevention

The four-point safety strategy (washing hands, doing a daily symptom check, socially distancing, and wearing a mask) is the practical strategy I recommend for reducing the individual and community risk of infection. While there are literally hundreds of things that we can try to do to reduce our risk in every conceivable or theoretical way, it is important for us—and most practical for us—to focus on these four practices and to do them exceptionally well.

Of course, it makes sense to optimize building ventilation, including opening windows if practical, and to decontaminate exposed surfaces on a regular basis. We should take these and other responsible measures whenever possible. Still, the higher priority is to wear a mask appropriately and to wash hands regularly. Similarly, I am not arguing against taking vitamins, meditating, taking herbal remedies, and taking steps to reduce stress and stay generally healthy and well. Behavioral health and wellness is extremely important during a pandemic, although not related to mask wearing for a safety purpose.

However, it's important to be wary of fake science news propagated over the internet, such as "experts" advocating for using vodka and vinegar as hand sanitizers, microwaving mail, gargling with seawater, relying on USB flash drives as protection, and so forth. Don't let all this bad advice and misinformation overwhelm and diminish your focus on reducing the largest portion of the risk that matters most. We should prioritize the four-point strategy above other possible ways to successfully diminish and control the pandemic.

In the following sections, I'll explain why these four practices are critical and how to carry them out effectively.

Washing Hands

When and why: Regardless of the source of the droplet exposure, hand-washing is one of the most important ways to prevent illness. Your hands become contaminated by droplets from the air as well as contaminated surfaces or objects or from touching your face or mouth. Germs may spread by preparing food or drinks or by blowing your nose or stifling a cough, or by shaking hands. Wash your hands *before* eating food, putting on a mask, or treating a wound. Wash your hands *after* cleaning another person, blowing your nose, or touching garbage or other contaminated surfaces. While many people have focused on environmental transmission by contaminated surfaces, this may account for as little as 6 percent of infections. Wash your hands at least five times per day, with possible additional benefit of up to 10 times per day.

How to wash effectively: Soap-and-water hand-washing removes more germs than hand sanitizers through the mechanical action and the destruction of lipids that form part of the coronavirus. When possible, use soap and water instead of a hand sanitizer, especially if your hands are visibly dirty or greasy. The disadvantages of hand-washing include a drying effect on hands, while hand sanitizers usually contain skin conditioners that may make them more tolerable. You do not need soap containing antibiotics, as these are not necessary for killing the virus. Follow these steps:

- Wet your hands with clean water and apply soap in a lather that covers all areas of your hands.

- Scrub your hands for 20 seconds (sing "Happy Birthday" or count)
- Rinse with clean, running water and dry with a clean towel or air dry.

Hand sanitizer is generally a good alternative to soap and water because it can be more conveniently applied outside of a restroom. It should contain at least 60 percent alcohol. This alcohol content should be indicated on the label of the hand sanitizer.

- Apply gel to hand in the amount recommended on the label, usually more than half a teaspoon or three milliliters. People often apply an insufficient amount.
- Rub your hands so that all surfaces are covered. Generally, this should take 20 seconds, similar to washing with soap and water.

Be careful not to let children use hand sanitizers without supervision, as this is a common cause of alcohol poisoning. Hand sanitizers are easy to use and are most effective in settings where hands are unlikely to become visibly dirty or greasy.

Daily Symptom Check

When and why: By mentally doing a symptom check every morning, you will avoid endangering others by leaving your home with symptoms. The MGB hospitals require employees to complete a symptom check on an app to verify that they have no symptoms before entering the hospital. By making a conscious mental note, you are more likely to really check your body for symptoms. You should leave work or go home if you develop symptoms at any point during the day or evening.

How: Symptoms may appear 2–14 days after exposure to the virus. People with any of the following symptoms may have COVID-19:

- Fever (100.4 degrees or higher; children 99.5 degrees orally) or chills; often with later onset
- New cough, other than due to preexisting allergy or asthma
- Shortness of breath or difficulty breathing
- Muscle or body aches, usually with other symptoms
- New loss of taste or smell
- Unexplained fatigue
- Sore throat
- Congestion or runny nose
- Nausea or vomiting, usually accompanying other symptoms
- Diarrhea, usually with other respiratory symptoms

None of these symptoms are unique to the coronavirus and may be commonly caused by the flu or other viruses or illnesses. While the loss of taste or smell is a striking symptom, it can be also attributed to other viral infections and causes. Some less-common symptoms and signs that may be associated with the coronavirus include purplish toes, streaky rashes, and conjunctivitis (pink eye).

If you develop any of these symptoms, it is important for you to call for clinical consultation, rather than physically visit an urgent care unit or hospital, unless it is an emergency. You will receive advice on whether it is necessary to visit in person or whether your symptoms can be handled through remote evaluation.

When you do a daily symptom check, it is important not to dismiss or ignore mild symptoms such as a sore throat or mild cough. It is possible to be highly infectious with mild symptoms because infectiousness is high during the initial part of the illness. Thus, it's important that individuals not go to work or to public areas if they're experiencing any symptoms.

Social Distancing

When and Why: Extra distance between yourself and others constitutes an additional protective effect, since droplets from exhalation without masking may fall within six feet. Furthermore, there's no guarantee that everyone will be constantly masked, making an additional layer of protection critical.

In either indoor or outdoor environments, social distancing is the physical distancing of six feet between each person who is not part of your household. Six feet is about two arm lengths. If both persons are wearing masks, then being closer than six feet for an incidental, short time is not a concern as long as there is no physical touching.

States impose density rules that limit the occupancy in buildings or the number allowed in a room as an additional protective effect. These social distancing and density rules protect against droplets being exhaled by asymptomatic infected people. These measures offer less protection when infected people are symptomatic; hence, it is important to stay home if you have symptoms.

How: Social distancing is difficult in a number of common situations, such as on transportation, at events or gatherings, while running errands, and dining at restaurants. Bars serving liquor represent especially high-risk situations.

- **Running errands:** Put on a mask before leaving your house or car. When standing in line, stay six feet apart and be mindful of the limit of the number of people allowed in a room or establishment.

- **Transportation:** The safest transportation involves traveling alone or with a small number of travelers. The most important rule if you are traveling with others is, of course, for everyone to wear masks when others are nearby. In addition, limit the number of people sitting side by side in a vehicle during extended rides. Select seats that leave some distance between you and others, understanding that greater distance is better, even if less than six feet. Avoid facing other passengers.
- **Events and gatherings:** It is better for everyone to be masked when at gatherings or events with a larger number of people. Situations involving eating as well as speaking loudly substantially increase the risk. The total number of people attending events should be kept as low as possible. Try to keep as much space as possible between yourself and others. Physical guides indicating spacing are helpful, including tape markings on floors and signs on walls to help keep people at least six feet apart.
- **Restaurants:** States have specific rules regarding the allowable density of people within a building space and whether indoor dining is allowed. Follow the spacing rules. Because it is not possible to wear masks while eating, respect for the six-foot rule is critically important. Limiting the number of diners at a table and eating outdoors when possible also reduce the risk.
- **Bars:** Visiting bars is a high-risk activity because eating and drinking don't allow for masking. Loud talking in close proximity adds to the risk, as does the possible loss of judgment from drinking alcohol.

Whenever possible, choose safer activities:

- Exercising outdoors is a good choice. Try to obey the six-foot rule between yourself and others, and decide whether you need to mask because of an inability to keep apart. Check on the density restrictions that may apply to parks or other recreational areas. Bring a mask to practice safe etiquette among those who are likely to be sensitive and aware of their health.
- Choose safer social activities such as contact by phone or social media. If visiting others in person, respect the six-foot rule and stick to small gatherings outdoors. Bring a mask as part of social etiquette, and be especially respectful of the elderly and those with medical vulnerabilities.

* * *

Masking is intertwined with these three basic practices and cannot be effectively practiced independently from them. (I will offer more detailed steps for effective masking in the following chapters.) All four practices together may success-fully protect us and others in our surrounding community. While masking has been shown to independently reduce risk, it also contributes to cohesive practice of the four-point strategy. We should consider washing our hands and checking for symptoms before putting on or taking off a mask. The sight of another person wearing a mask reminds us to keep a reasonable distance, and studies show that those who wear masks regularly are more likely to practice social distancing. Masking also helps reinforce other safety practices, including not touching one's face or mouth. Thus, masking must be an integrated part of this multipronged strategy of prevention.

CHAPTER 3

Universal Masking in a Culture of Community Safety

Universal mask-wearing is most likely to succeed in a culture of community safety. Such a culture is based on shared core values and behaviors that emphasize a continuous commitment to safety over competing goals. It gives us a workable alternative to being locked down in fear or reopening our social and business activities without reasonable precautions. In short, an acceptance of the importance of masks within a culture committed to safety can allow us to move forward confidently by reopening in a predictable and deliberate way consistent with rigorous medical science.

Universal mask-wearing is not a silver bullet that will halt the pandemic in its tracks, nor is it a complete cure in itself. Rather, it is a public health tool that needs to be integrated into the social fabric of safety promotion that protects the whole community. An inclusive and cohesive culture is required to continually remind individuals of the responsibility to embrace this community-wide safety strategy. Safe behavior must become part of our daily individual and group consciousness, from taking a moment each day to check ourselves for symptoms, to washing our hands at least five times daily, to avoiding crowded indoor environments, particularly when eating, and—of course—wearing a mask.

This chapter outlines what such a culture of safety looks like as well as the steps individuals, businesses, and communities can take to promote it. I start with an exploration of safety in hospitals, where the concept of a culture of safety originated.

The Culture of Safety in Hospitals

Since the 1990s, hospitals have been at the vanguard of developing and maintaining a culture of safety. This cultural movement was initiated by the Institute of Medicine's call for accountability of hospitals to prevent medical errors, which at the time killed more people than car accidents or breast cancer—between 44,000 to 98,000 Americans each year. The Institute of Medicine attributed the high number of patient deaths to the decentralized and fragmented nature of health-care delivery. Its report in 2000 called for the protection of patients based on their right to freedom from accidental injury. Since then, hospitals have been required to develop programs consistent with reducing preventable adverse events, including hospital-acquired infections.

Hospitals have developed a number of methods to minimize preventable harm to patients, such as supporting a "safety climate" that encourages and enables individuals to contribute to identifying medical errors and reducing them. This has led to concrete safety protocols, such as the development and utilization of safety checklists to prevent errors in operating rooms and inpatient units. Thus, it is not surprising that hospitals developed safety measures to protect patients and health-care workers from the coronavirus based on their existing culture of safety.

At the Mass General Brigham (MGB) hospital system, universal masking of both employees and patients is now central to its culture of safety, aptly named the Safe Care Commitment to both patients and employees. Indeed, this Safe Care Commitment incorporates the four-point strategy discussed in the last chapter based on key CDC guidance. At the MGB, we have emphasized the importance of communicating this four-point strategy at a centralized as well as a hospital-based level. We provide evidence-based, relevant information and data to those working within the hospital system. These communications specifically emphasize the importance of personal symptom checks, wearing appropriate personal protective equipment in special contexts such as aerosolizing procedures, and respecting the need for social distancing in work break rooms and while eating. Our hospital system has also adopted two important programs to provide systematic support for our culture of safety: a mandatory flu vaccination program and coronavirus testing for hospital workers based on consistent medical criteria.

Flu Vaccination Programs
Our hospital system has adopted a mandatory program of flu vaccination for all employees and non-employed visitors to the clinical affiliates. It is based on the notion that patients should expect that whomever cares for them in the hospital is vaccinated to reduce the risk of becoming exposed to the flu. While other hospitals have compulsory vaccination programs for this reason, our hospital requirement is unusual in that it applies to literally "all" employees, including those who work in purely administrative buildings in nonclinical activities, such as finance or human resources. Our mandatory vaccination program also includes outside visitors such as vendors providing food services or visiting for business-related purposes.

So why do we vaccinate nonclinical staff in buildings far removed from our hospital and clinic sites? Our hospital leadership is committed to the principle that all employees have an obligation to serve as role models for our patients and community. The CDC recommends flu vaccines for everyone six months of age and older with only rare medical exceptions. The medical contraindications to the flu vaccine include having a serious allergic reaction to the flu vaccine or past medical history of Guillain-Barre syndrome, a rare form of paralysis after vaccination. Both medical contraindications are uncommon, and these risks for the general population are substantially outweighed by the protection provided by flu vaccinations. Employees with medical contraindications to flu vaccines are exempted from the requirement with proper medical documentation. However, they are required to wear masks in clinical areas during flu season.

During the current coronavirus pandemic, many of our nonhospital employees are working remotely and may not set foot into any MGB building. Nevertheless, we are still requiring them to be vaccinated because of the high importance of extra protection during this coronavirus pandemic. Because flu symptoms may be identical to those of a coronavirus infection, it is important to reduce the need to be tested for the coronavirus. Having a flu shot reduces the possibility of having to visit a medical provider because of illness and avoids hospitalization from the flu. Because it is also possible to be coinfected with the flu and coronavirus, it is critically important that most people get vaccinated for the flu, ideally early in the fall season, as explained in more detail in chapter 6.

The Importance of Employee Health Services for Organizations

Shortly after the first coronavirus case appeared in Massachusetts, the MGB system established a service center staffed by nurse clinicians that provided coronavirus-related services to its workers. This sudden expansion of clinical occupational health services represented another first-in-the-country development for the Harvard Medical School-affiliated system. Given the unprecedented demand by hospital workers for coronavirus-related services, its clinical staffing tripled within two weeks. The service center created a large-scale telehealth system that provided medical advice, referrals, and testing for its 78,000 employees. Thus, when testing became available at the six MGB sites, employees were able to have direct and timely access to critical diagnostic and medical information services.

An important service provided by the service center is providing medical advice based on CDC criteria about returning to work. A hospital employee with a confirmed test for coronavirus and with symptoms is kept out of work for a minimum of 14 days from the first appearance of symptoms and until at least three days after recovery and resolution of symptoms. Hospitals may also follow testing-based criteria that require negative testing before an employee is allowed to return to work. These return-to-work criteria differ from those for workers outside hospital settings, who have a lower risk of infecting vulnerable immunocompromised patients. If you are not a hospital worker, you may return to work 10 days after the first appearance of symptoms as long as you have been fever-free for 24 hours without the use of fever-reducing medications and other symptoms are improving.

Financial support by employers is another important means of creating stronger incentives to reduce community risk. For example, an important benefit for MGB employees is "COVID pay," which allows symptomatic employees to continue receiving regular pay without using earned time off if promptly tested and kept out of work until test results are received. If the test result is negative, COVID pay ceases. If, however, the test result is positive, affected employees are provided with COVID pay for up to 30 days depending on the time of recovery. This pay benefit encourages workers to be promptly tested and to stay away from work if symptoms develop. This ensures patients and other workers avoid exposure to a potentially infectious individual.

Society at large has an opportunity to learn from the hospital experience in developing a culture of safety. First, a commitment to the four-point safety strategy must be incorporated into our social fabric. We need to develop shared competencies and safe behavior by following a responsible science-based approach to living in the coronavirus pandemic. In short, we need to adopt the approach that has kept hospital workers safe in a potentially dangerous environment. The science tells us that masks work, and that the way to avoid staying mired in a lockdown is to put the four-point strategy front and center in our public health management of the pandemic.

Developing a Safety Culture That Supports Reopenings by States

Countries that have successfully managed and controlled the pandemic have imposed mandates for the public to wear masks in public settings. I describe research studies in chapter 9 that demonstrate the association between adoption of these mandates by countries and states and improved management of the pandemic spread. The federal government should provide guidance and regulatory support to help states reinforce mask mandates when necessary to better control the rate of new infections. States can effectively manage and control the pandemic by tracking the rate of mask usage in "hot spot" communities and other key areas. The degree of public participation in universal mask-wearing should inform the states' determination of the timing and pace of reopening activities for public spaces and businesses. States can consider a phased reopening approach that bases allowed activity levels on the prevalence of mask usage through systematic and standard-ized surveys in key communities. Public face mask usage has been reliably tracked in cities, states, and regions.[1] If phased reopening activities are linked to a higher prevalence of mask usage, municipalities and individuals will be encouraged to increase mask usage.

Like any public health or medical intervention, universal masking has definite limitations. For example, masking isn't feasible while eating, which means there is increased risk if there is close socializing. For this reason, reopening bars is highly risky. Restaurants must set up tables out of doors to the extent possible and allow indoor dining only with sufficient social distancing. Thus, before states adopt the last phase of reopening that opens up bars and regular indoor dining, they must reach a stable and very low number of newly identified cases, since masking won't be adequate in these situations.

On the other hand, masking may reduce risk effectively in other high-risk situations. States should require mask-wearing for passengers on public transportation, for example. To con-trol against further infectious spread within infected house-holds, public health agencies need to promote the four-point strategy through home visits. State enforcement of these rules promotes a shared cultural understanding of the limits to con-trolling infection when masks cannot be used and the value of enforcing mask requirements more strictly in specific, high-risk situations.

A masking policy may be a more effective public health tool than quarantine measures to control the spread of infec-tion from states with higher risk. While quarantines have a definite role in public health, it is difficult for governments to effectively enforce travel restrictions between states. It is

1   J. Hatzius, D. Struyven, and I. Rosenberg. Face masks and GDP, Goldman Sachs Research. June 29, 2020. https://www.golmansachs.com/insights/pages/face-masks -and-gdp.html

impossible for governments or employers to know when people engage in personal travel to higher-risk areas in other states and thus should be quarantined. Because masking is visible and effective, especially in reducing the infectivity by asymptomatic persons, it may prove to be advantageous for governments to rely more on masking mandates than on self-enforced quarantines.

Another important element of maintaining a culture of safety in hospitals is not blaming individuals who make mistakes, while encouraging a reduction in medical errors through learning and systematic changes. We should encourage individuals to promote proper mask-wearing, but avoid the negative, counterproductive consequences of being rude to those who may forget or not fully appreciate the importance of this safety approach. Similarly, individuals should not be upset or confront others in situations where there is a perceived incidental invasion of the six-foot safety buffer as long as those involved are wearing masks. Mask-wearing should promote better social relations, not increased hostility.

Businesses should also make it easier for visitors to point out a friendly "please wear a mask" sign and make masks available, as well as promote hand-washing or antiseptic hand rubs. We should adopt the shared belief that wearing a mask is a friendly and healthy way to live. The mask must become a talisman of care for others, just as it reassures patients of their safety when worn by those in the OR and elsewhere in hospital settings. Conversely, those who forget or improperly wear masks should appreciate others pointing this out in a nonjudgmental way, rather than react to this as a criticism or invasion of privacy. In the end, the effectiveness of masking comes down to developing a shared ethic to support and protect each other and ourselves.

CHAPTER 4

Mask Types, Wearing, and Care

In the coronavirus era, a fundamental principle of public safety is wearing a mask in public areas—even wearing a lower-quality mask, such as a bandana or handkerchief, is better than no mask at all. The CDC and other public health agencies recommend cloth masks for public use and prefer to reserve medical-grade masks (surgical masks and N95 respirators) for health-care workers to avoid shortages. Health-care workers, who spend extended periods in high-risk environments, rely on surgical masks and in some especially high-risk areas, N-95 respirators, face shields, and additional personal protective equipment.

A standard cloth mask is a double-layer mask made of cotton in a tight weave. The natural fabric acts as a filter that diminishes droplet spread because its irregular physical microstructure blocks the small droplets. Another excellent material for masks is polypropylene fiber, which is used in surgical masks and N95 respirators. This fiber has an electrostatic charge that causes viral particles to cling to it.

A recent development is the marketing of clear masks with plastic panels that allow one's face to be more visible. Further scientific testing should be done to evaluate this promising alternative, since it relies on a different approach to limiting droplet spread. While the CDC has not yet offered guidance about the effectiveness of such masks, it recommends them to support those who may be hearing impaired.

You've probably heard a lot of conflicting information about masks, their use, and their effectiveness in the past few months. In the sections below, I will answer some of the most common questions I've fielded from patients, colleagues, and community members.

What type of cloth mask is desirable?

The CDC recommends cloth masks for public use. The fibers of cloth masks block viral particles from traveling a longer distance. They also filter droplets and reduce their spread. The most widely recommended material for cloth masks is 100 percent cotton, since the natural fibers in cotton tend to have an irregular physical structure that blocks particles, unlike synthetic fibers. Hybrid combinations containing polyester, cotton, chiffon, silk, flannel, spandex, and others may also be adequate filters. A recent study rated a three-layer cotton-polypropylene-cotton mask as a highly effective cloth mask. Cotton should provide a comfortable layer close to your face.

If you are choosing cotton, choose a fabric with a tight weave. You may check on this by holding the fabric to the light. If you see individual fibers, the weave is not sufficiently tight. Multilayering with two to three layers is another good feature to look for because of the increased filtering it offers. Pleats or folds allow expansion of the mask and reduce the chance of viral transmission through gaps at the sides.

Can I make my own cloth mask?

Yes! Many websites offer instructions and patterns for home-made masks, including the website for the CDC, which I provide here: https://www.cdc.gov/coronavirus/2019-ncov/prevent-getting-sick/how-to-make-cloth-face-covering.html.

Use heavier cotton material, such as quilting cotton or cotton sheets with a tight weave. You can also use cotton material from sheets or a T-shirt.

How do I put on a mask correctly?

- Wash your hands before putting on a mask.
- Place it over your nose and mouth and secure it under the chin by using ear loops or ties.
- Check to make sure that the mask is snug against your face.
- Check your breathing to make sure that you are comfortable.

How should a cloth mask fit?

Cloth masks should fit snugly and comfortably over the nose and mouth, with no gaps on the sides (gaps can reduce filtration efficiency by over 60 percent). If needed, adjust the elastic ear loops or ties to hold the mask close to your face. Your mask should not be tight or uncomfortable.

How breathable should a cloth mask be?

You should be able to breathe without restriction. The tradeoff is that more breathable masks have increased porosity, which means reduced filtering. However, it is important that breathing be comfortable to allow mask use to be maximized. Masks made of two to three layers of permeable fabric are generally breathable while still effective in filtering.

How do I avoid fogging my glasses when wearing a cloth mask?

If you wear glasses, look for a mask with a bendable border at the top so you can mold the mask to fit over the bridge of your nose to create a snug fit. Wear your glasses over the mask to prevent fogging.

Do beards cause a problem with fitting cloth masks and attracting viruses?
There is no evidence that shaving beards will help prevent infection by the coronavirus. However, beards are not recommended for health-care workers who need to wear N95 respirators, which must be tightly fitted. But because cloth and surgical masks fit more loosely than respirators, there should generally be no problem wearing them over beards as long as one can maintain a sufficiently snug fit.

What is the best way to take off a cloth mask?
- Release the ear loops or untie the strings.
- Hold the mask only by the loops or ties.
- If you are transporting the mask, fold it so the contaminated outside is folded inward against itself. Avoid touching this side of the mask. Put it into a clean paper bag.
- Place the mask in the washing machine or wash with warm water and soap.
- Do not touch your eyes, nose, or mouth. Wash your hands after removing the mask.

How should I store a cloth mask?
The best way to store a cloth mask when you are carrying it around is in a clean paper bag.

How often should I wash my cloth mask?
Wash masks daily in the washing machine with detergent or by hand with soap and hot water. Use a mask only if it is dry.

Are gaiters an effective type of mask?
Neck-gaiter masks are often made of synthetic fabric and wrap around, so there is less air escaping from the sides. Studies of their effectiveness are limited and show mixed results, with

some controversy over their testing evaluation techniques. A gaiter may be a better filter if folded to provide two layers. There is some concern, however, about the potential accumulation of droplets in areas likely to be touched.

What about the value and effectiveness of masks with see-through plastic panels?
Clear masks are becoming popular, especially among children. However, the scientific data on the safety efficacy of clear masks is still limited. While the CDC recommends clear masks as support for the deaf, who would otherwise have difficulty receiving communication, it has not yet offered guidance for general public use. Since the plastic panel does not allow filtration in front of the mouth and nose, further investigation of the effectiveness of this type of mask in reducing droplet spread would be helpful. Some clear masks rely on silicone and plastic covering filters for this purpose. It may also be important to consider breathability, ease of cleaning, and possible fogging issues.

Should I use cloth masks with a pocket for a filter?
No strong scientific evidence supports an increased benefit of this feature, but this is still being studied. Probably the best filter is polypropylene, a material used in surgical masks, which has an electrostatic charge that provides a static electric cling to droplets. Other filters include HEPA filters or tissue. If you use a filter, keep it in the pocket between layers of fabric to avoid breathing in fibers from the filter. Do not use coffee filters, which are hard to breathe through; you will end up breathing around the filter rather than through it. Do not use a filter if it makes it difficult for you to breathe.

Is a face shield as effective as a cloth mask?
A face shield is a rigid piece of plastic that is attached to a headband that extends down over the chin. Some people

prefer them over masks because the face is visible and they are more comfortable to wear. However, a face shield by itself may provide less protection than a mask because unfiltered air can still flow around the sides and bottom. If everyone masks and is able to socially distance at six feet, there is no need for a face shield. If, however, social distancing is not possible, then wearing both a mask and a face shield may increase protection. Scientific data on the effectiveness of public wearing of face shields along with masks is limited.

What about goggles?
While it is possible to become infected through your eyes from droplets, there is no public health guidance that recommends that the general public wear goggles. However, the CDC recommends that health-care workers wear eye protection when in close contact with patients in areas with moderate to substantial community transmission, and health-care workers wear goggles or face shields along with masks when caring for patients infected with coronavirus. Eye protection may be appropriate outside the health-care realm in certain situations, such as a hairstylist working face-to-face with customers. Eyeglasses may provide only limited protection because of the space between the glasses and the face.

How are surgical masks used?
Surgical masks are becoming more widely available, although the CDC recommends that they be reserved for health-care workers. Like cloth masks, they fit more loosely than N95 respirators. Higher-quality surgical masks are made of polypropylene fiber, rather than paper, which provides an electrostatic charge that captures viral particles. This composition also makes surgical masks more breathable. Surgical masks may block outward transmission of respiratory viruses up to three times better than cloth masks, although some studies

show that well-made multilayered cotton masks are nearly as effective. Surgical masks are not washable, and should be discarded when they become dirty or damaged.

How is an N-95 respirator different than a mask?

N95 respirators are designed to protect both the wearer and others nearby because they filter 95 percent or more of airborne particles as small as 3 microns. They are made of layers of polypropylene fibers whose static electricity traps both incoming and outgoing droplets. Supplies of N95 respirators are limited, so hospitals reserve them for clinicians whose work exposes them to high levels of airborne coronavirus. N95 respirators are designed to fit tightly around the nose and mouth. Health-care workers are fit tested and provided medical clearance before being allowed to use N95 respirators. A seal check should be done at regular intervals. They are less comfortable to wear than masks because of their tighter fit.

What about KN95 respirators?

KN95 respirators are made by Chinese manufacturers under regulation by their government. They are supposed to work like N95 respirators and filter at least 95 percent of small particles. However, there are many fakes, and unlike N95 respirators, their quality and functionality are not consistent.

Why should I avoid masks with exhalation valves?

Some masks and N95 respirators have exhalation valves that make it easier to breathe out. They were originally manufactured for use in industrial construction and intended to protect wearers against dust exposure rather than infectious disease prevention. Their valves release unfiltered air, meaning they don't block viral transmission to others and are thus ineffective for infectious disease protection.

CHAPTER 5

When to Wear a Mask

Masking must become universal if we wish to control the pandemic. Face masks should be worn in public areas where there is the possibility of coming in close contact with others. It is probably safe to walk or jog unmasked when no one else is around. However, if you happen to approach or pass others in public, face covering is the primary means of protecting them from the invisible droplets you expel while breathing.

As an example, the universal masking policy at hospitals relies on everyone putting on a mask at the building entrance and wearing it throughout the day. The only narrow exception to this restriction is when one is eating. Many of the infections transmitted at hospitals with universal masking occur during work breaks, when masks slip down or are taken off. In August, a hospital in the western part of Massachusetts experienced an outbreak that affected 14 patients and 26 employees. It started when a hospital employee returned to work after traveling to a hotspot state. The employee exposed others in a hospital break room, where masks were not being worn.

This chapter answers common questions about safe mask-wearing in a number of common situations. My goal is to offer commonsense, practical solutions and information so you can better understand your own role in public safety and assess your personal risk level when choosing your activities.

Why isn't it safe to be around people who appear healthy, don't have symptoms, and are not wearing a mask?
Almost half of coronavirus infections come from exposure to people without symptoms. Up to 30–40 percent of those infected do not manifest any symptoms. Those who are infected and do not have symptoms have the same amount of viral shedding as those with symptoms. Additionally, people can become highly infectious a day or two before they start experiencing symptoms. Furthermore, it's unlikely someone next to you with a mild sore throat or headache will inform you of these potential coronavirus symptoms. It is the pervasiveness and invisibility of the coronavirus that makes it highly infectious.

Why is wearing a mask especially important for protecting those who are medically vulnerable?
Another reason for universal mask-wearing is that we can't pick and choose whom we expose based on medical risk. Those who are especially vulnerable and for whom infection poses a significant risk of severe illness, hospitalization, and poor medical outcomes include those with underlying medical conditions such as chronic lung disease, an immunocompromised state, serious heart conditions, sickle cell disease, and type 2 diabetes. These conditions can't be readily identified by sight. Furthermore, a large proportion of our population has more visibly identifiable risk factors, such as advanced age or obesity: Twenty-one percent of our population is over the age of 60 years, and 30 percent has a body mass index of 30 or greater. Thus, it is important to wear a mask when around anyone in public areas, since the vulnerable may be impossible to identify by sight, and those with significant risk factors constitute a large proportion of the general population.

Who should not wear a mask?
Masks should be worn whenever possible. However, a few narrowly defined populations should not wear them:

- Those who have trouble breathing when wearing a mask
- Those unable to remove a mask without assistance (such as those with physical or mental disabilities or those who are incapacitated or unconscious)
- Children younger than two years old
- Those engaged in an activity that will wet their masks (e.g., swimming)
- Those engaged in an activity in which a mask may cause difficulty breathing (e.g., running)
- Those working in conditions where a mask may increase occupational safety risk (e.g., straps caught in machinery) or when a mask may contribute to heat-related illness

If you are unable to wear a mask, it is important to reduce risk to a maximum extent by social distancing and being vigilant about hand-washing and symptom monitoring.

What are the riskiest environments?
The highest-risk environments are those in which you are surrounded by many people not wearing masks and unable to socially distance. These also include settings where people may be speaking loudly, singing, or vigorously exhaling. Such settings may include bars, large concerts, and gyms. Risk increases based on the number of people, amount of social distancing and degree of proximity, number of people wearing masks, number of people who are not part of your household, indoor space, and degree of community transmission.

Should I wear a mask when I go to a restaurant?
If you dine out, it is safest to go with those in your household since it is difficult to socially distance while seated. While no one expects you to wear a mask while eating, it is important to wear a mask when you are headed to the restaurant. Check the restaurant's website to ensure that it observes safety guidelines, including maintaining social distancing and controlling the density of customers and tables, having their staff wear masks, and offering outdoor dining. Self-parking is preferable to valet parking. Wash your hands before and after your meal. When you take off your mask while seated, store it in a plastic or paper bag to keep it clean. To avoid contaminating your hands, take off your mask by the ear straps, rather than touching the fabric covering your face. Wear a mask when away from your table and in any entryway or waiting area. Wearing a mask when you are near others should be part of our social etiquette. Consider choosing a mask with an interesting design and color that reflects how you want to look and feel and incorporate it into your social interactions with others.

What about attending social events or gatherings?
You should weigh the risks of attending social gatherings, including weddings and other social events. Take into account your own medical vulnerability and that of others, the size of the gathering, and the rate of community transmission. If you decide to participate, it is critical that you follow the four-point safety protocol. Stay at home if you have even mild symptoms. Check with the event's organizer about how they intend to keep the event safe. Prioritize outdoor gatherings with a smaller number of guests over indoor events with large crowds that may be talking loudly or singing. Limit your physical contact and do not hug or shake hands. Respect social distancing to the extent possible. Avoid contact with

shared surfaces and avoid any self-serve food. Wash your hands before, during, and after the event. One possible way for event organizers to emphasize the acceptability and importance of mask-wearing is by providing colorful and interesting masks to all guests.

Is going to a hair salon or barbershop safe?
Getting one's hair done may be reasonably safe if everyone is masked. Recall the observational study in chapter 1 of the two hairstylists in Springfield, Missouri and their 139 clients—both stylists had the coronavirus, but because both they and their clients were masked, none of their clients contracted it. Hairstylists may optimize their safety by wearing both masks and face shields.

Is it safe to visit a hospital or clinic?
Yes, it is reasonably safe to see a medical provider if you comply with the facility's safety policy, and it is important not to forgo necessary and important medical evaluations and treatments. Hospitals have now adopted universal masking policies along with other safety measures. However, clinical services by telemedicine further decrease the risk to patients and health-care workers while making care more convenient. If you have a fever or infectious illness, it is better to check with the clinical facility first before visiting, unless it is an urgent situation.

What about staying as a guest in a hotel?
When staying in a hotel, wear a mask except when in your hotel room. You should wear a mask in the lobby and other common areas. Many hotels offer contact-free options for routine interactions, such as online reservations and check-in, mobile room keys, and contactless payment. All staff should wear masks, and hotels are required to meet other state

safety requirements, including Plexiglas barriers and physical arrangements that reinforce social distancing. If you use an elevator, maintain social distance as much as possible by standing in a corner of the elevator and not entering an elevator in which the corner areas are already occupied by those outside your household.

What are the masking requirements for flying?
All commercial airlines have mandatory masking for those over two years of age. Check with the individual airline regarding specific issues. Most airlines do not permit face shields as substitutes for masks and ban masks with exhaust valves, vents, or mesh.

What about gyms and fitness centers?
These are potentially high-risk environments because of the indoor environment and the more forcible exhalation associated with exercise, along with the difficulty of wearing a mask during exercise. If possible, choose to exercise outdoors and in less-crowded environments. If you decide to use a gym or fitness center, check if the facility offers online or phone reservations to ensure you can socially distance. You should also confirm that the gym offers physical facilities that reinforce social distancing, outdoor workout options, or virtual gym classes. Equipment must be cleaned and disinfected regularly. Also, consider wearing a mask when stretching, walking, or doing yoga or other low-intensity exercise.

Do I need a mask for recreational jogging or running?
You may have difficulty wearing a mask during highly intensive exercise such as jogging because of the decreased breathability of masks, so with proper social distancing, you can run without a mask. You should consider running outside and maintaining a physical distance from others, rather than running

in a pack. Also, keep in mind that as you run, you are forcibly exhaling and hence sending invisible droplets a greater distance than usual from your nose and mouth.

What about swimming?
Do not wear a mask while swimming. Masks are difficult to breathe through when wet, and there is no scientific evidence that the coronavirus can spread through water during recreational swimming. Since masks should not be worn, it is important to comply as closely as possible with the other safety practices, namely washing hands, social distancing, symptom monitoring, and wearing a mask when not in the water. Pool operators should ensure the availability of supplies to support healthy hygiene, including soap, hand sanitizer, and clean towels. Touched surfaces should be regularly decontaminated.

How long do I have to be exposed to an unmasked infected person to consider getting tested?
The CDC definition of a significant exposure event in a hospital setting occurs when an individual (without a mask or eye protection) is within six feet of an infected person not wearing a mask, such as a fellow worker or patient, for 15 minutes. If a person has been significantly exposed for 15 or more minutes in this situation, then careful symptom monitoring is important for the following 14 days, and testing is recommended within 2 to 10 days after the identified exposure. Contact tracing may also be recommended in such situations. This approach emphasizes the importance of continual mask-wearing in public spaces, particularly when social distancing cannot be maintained.

CHAPTER 6

Masking in Households and for Children

The previous chapters explored mask-wearing in public settings when you're around people outside your household. However, masking also has a special role in the home if a member of your household becomes infected with coronavirus. This chapter also addresses common questions about mask-wearing by children.

Households

Do members of the same household share a similar risk of infection since they live in the same home environment? How does this affect the approach to masking?

Household members share a similar risk among themselves because it is difficult to socially distance while at home, and you are normally not expected to wear masks inside the home. Thus, household members are not ordinarily expected to socially distance from each other when in public spaces. If a member of the household is older or has a medical condition that puts them at increased risk for severe illness from the coronavirus, the rest of the household should try to protect that person by behaving in public areas as if they themselves are at higher risk.

What if a household member becomes ill with the coronavirus?

The risk of infection transmission between household members is high in the household environment. The ill person should stay in their own room or space and maintain social distancing from the others in the household. Any household members at higher risk due to age or medical conditions should be kept away from the ill person. It is important for the household to isolate the sick member and follow the directions from your medical provider and quarantine directions from the state or local health department:

- The sick household member should wear a mask when around others. Masks are effective in reducing household transmission.[1] If a surgical-type mask is available, the sick member should wear it.
- Only one person in the household should take care of the person who is sick. The caregiver should wear a mask and gloves when in the area where the sick member is staying and clean only where necessary to limit contact with the sick person. The caregiver should also minimize contact with others in the household and consider wearing a mask in their presence.
- High-touch areas of the home should be disinfected daily. Household members should avoid sharing phones, dishes, or bedding with the ill member. Ideally, the ill member should use a separate bathroom from others in the household.

---

1   Wang Y, Tian H, Zhang L, et al. Reduction of secondary transmission of SARS-CoV-2 in households by face mask use, disinfection and social distancing: a cohort study in Beijing, China. *BMJ Glob Health*. 2020;5(5):e002794. doi:10.1136/bmjgh-2020-002794

The masked caregiver should be the only one to bring food to the sick person. Laundry for the ill person should also be kept separate.
- Visitors to the home should be discouraged.

Who needs to be quarantined if a household member becomes ill with the coronavirus?

People who have been in close contact with someone who has coronavirus, including household members, must be quarantined. Close contact is defined as any of the following:

- Within six feet of someone infected with coronavirus for a total of 15 minutes or more.
- You provided care at home to someone ill with coronavirus.
- You had direct physical contact with the person.
- You shared eating or drinking utensils.
- The infected person sneezed, coughed, or got respiratory droplets on you.

Quarantine for coronavirus is defined as isolation from others for a minimum of 14 days following the last contact with the ill person. Those under quarantine must stay home and monitor themselves for symptoms for a minimum of 14 days. They must also follow directions from their medical provider and their state or local health department.

If a member of your household becomes ill with the coronavirus, it is likely that all household members will need to be quarantined for a minimum of 14 days after their last close contact with the ill household member, since household members typically don't wear masks at home.

When can home isolation and masking within the household be discontinued for persons infected with the coronavirus?
Infected individuals and household members can end their quarantine under the following conditions:

- After at least 10 days from the symptom onset, and
- At least 24 hours since resolution of fever without the use of fever-reducing medications and
- Other symptoms have improved.

Notice that it is possible for an infected person to end their isolation earlier than other household members because of the possibility that the other household members may have been infected from their exposure to the original infected person. If the infected person has had a severe illness or is immunocompromised, their medical provider may extend their isolation for 20 days or more.

Is it necessary for household members to receive a flu shot in the fall, given the protective impact of universal masking?
Yes—it is especially important to be vaccinated for the flu with the risk of coronavirus circulating in the community. Getting a flu shot will likely substantially reduce the risk of developing flu symptoms, which can be indistinguishable from those for the coronavirus. While wearing masks will help reduce the risk of flu, another virus propagated by droplet spread, everyone over the age of six months should receive a flu shot unless they have a medical contraindication. The flu itself is a dangerous infection, and there is a serious concern that hospitals will become overwhelmed with admissions if people are not vaccinated for the flu.

Is it possible for pets to be infected with the coronavirus? Should pets wear masks?

A small number of pet cats and dogs have been infected with the virus after contact with infected people. Other types of animals that have been infected by the coronavirus include lions, tigers, and minks. This is based on very limited data, and there is no evidence that animals have a significant role in spreading the coronavirus to people, as the pandemic is driven by person-to-person transmission. The risk of infection from pets is thought to be low. Nevertheless, the recommendation is to protect your pets and service animals from exposure to infected people or sick animals. Do not put masks on animals as they may risk suffocation.

Children

Should children wear masks in public?

Yes, children over the age of two years should wear masks in public areas just as adults do. Children under age five may require close supervision to ensure they're wearing their masks safely. Based on limited available data, children under the age of 10 appear to be less likely to be infected than adults and are more likely to be asymptomatic. Children under the age of five with mild to moderate infection have higher amounts of coronavirus in their nasopharynx than older children and adults. However, it is unclear whether this makes them more infectious. There is limited data from small studies suggesting that children are more likely to become infected by adults than be a source of infection. This limited data tends to show that children are not the major infective driver of the pandemic, but there is substantial uncertainty given the limited data size and our lack of evidence since schools were closed early in the pandemic.

Are there children who should not wear masks?
Yes, children who should not wear masks include the following:

- Those under the age of two years
- Unsupervised children who may choke on mask if left on their own
- Those with difficulty breathing because of asthma or other respiratory conditions
- Those who are incapacitated or otherwise unable to remove a mask without assistance

Are face shields a good alternative to masks for children under the age of two years?
No, for safety reasons, neither face shields nor masks are recommended for children under the age of two. The CDC does not generally recommend face shields for everyday use because of the lack of sufficient data on their effectiveness.

What about children using clear masks?
Clear masks have a plastic panel that keeps the mouth and face visible. However, the data for their efficacy is limited, and the CDC has not made any recommendations for clear masks for general use. It has, however, recommended clear masks for teachers and caregivers of children with hearing disabilities. The CDC's approach suggests that we need a practical approach to masking and to understand that the central goal is to achieve universal masking.

Should children wear masks at school?
Yes, it is important that children wear masks when attending school and follow the four-point safety strategy that includes frequent hand-washing, daily symptom monitoring, and social distancing. Children are less likely to become infected than adults and less likely to experience severe disease, although a

rare subset do become seriously ill with a multisystem inflammatory syndrome.

How can I encourage my child to wear a mask?

Getting younger children to wear masks might take time. We need to be patient, reassuring, and allow them time to get used to the new experience. Some children may find it scary at first not to be able to see a person's whole face. Here are some suggestions for making your child comfortable with masking:

- Explain that masks are important for protecting others and perhaps themselves. Teach your child about the infectivity of the coronavirus.
- Give children time to practice wearing masks before they wear them outside of the home. Teach them how to put their masks on and how to take them off.
- Encourage children to make and decorate their masks. You might also allow masks to be part of their play so they will become a more normal part of their life.

What should I consider when choosing a mask for a child?

In general, choosing a mask for a child is similar to choosing a mask for an adult. It is important to find a mask that fits snugly and comfortably so the child is not constantly adjusting it or touching their face. It should also be washable. Ideally, it should have a double layer of breathable fabric such as dense cotton and attach comfortably with ear loops or straps. Your child should be able to breathe easily. To encourage wearing, you may let your child choose a mask he or she finds attractive.

Should my child attend youth and summer camps?
Responsible parents need to carefully assess their child's risk.
There is less risk under the following conditions:
- Staff and children wear masks
- There are smaller groups of children
- There is close supervision and social distancing is practiced as much as possible with no sharing of objects
- The camp is focused on outdoor activity
- Participants are from the local area
- It's not an overnight camp

CHAPTER 7

Adverse Effects and Discomfort

Masks, especially cloth masks, are generally well-tolerated and not associated with serious adverse effects. The two most common complaints from wearers are about skin problems and breathability. To complicate the issue, myths have circulated widely in social media about claims that masks cause dangerous oxygen depletion (hypoxia) and carbon dioxide poisoning (hypercapnia). But in reality, the most serious risks associated with masks come from violence between strangers who disagree about masking.

In this chapter, I will address some of the common concerns about masks—from how to minimize any discomfort from wearing them to understanding the facts and fiction behind some popular beliefs about mask-wearing.

Are there medical reasons not to wear a cloth mask?
If you are having genuine difficulty breathing while wearing a cloth mask, you should consult with a clinician. Since cloth masks are porous and should not fit tightly, unlike N95 respirators, it is unusual for them to cause such severe distress that mask-wearing is contraindicated. Even those with asthma or chronic lung conditions may often still wear cloth masks safely after examination by a clinician. Other reasons for not wearing a mask include being under two years of age or having

a disability that makes it difficult to remove a mask. Some behavioral disabilities also make it difficult to keep a mask on.

What kind of mask should I choose if I am concerned about developing skin problems?

On the inside of the mask, it may be helpful to have a natural, smooth, soft, and breathable material such as tightly woven cotton. Cotton is particularly desirable if you have acne or oily skin. The mask should fit snugly, but not tightly.

What can I do to reduce the likelihood of skin problems?

There are a number of easy steps you can take to reduce the chance of skin irritation.

- Wash your face daily with a mild, fragrance-free cleanser.
- Apply a moisturizer before and after wearing a mask to reduce irritation associated with dry skin. If you have chapped lips, apply petroleum jelly.
- Avoid applying makeup to areas of your face covered by your mask.
- Wash your mask daily to remove oils and skin cells that collect on the mask. Use soap and water or a detergent that does not leave residual odor or irritate your skin.
- Contact a dermatologist if you develop an irritation or rash that does not resolve within a short time. If you have an underlying skin condition, such as acne or rosacea, continue your current treatment.

How can I stop irritation associated with elastic ear loops?

The elastic ear loops on your mask may cause irritation behind your ears. You can obtain masks that don't rely on elastic ear loops to stay in place, but use clips instead. Some call these "ear savers." You may also use masks with tie-on straps.

What can I do if I don't like the decrease in breathability?
It may take time to learn to breathe comfortably in your mask, just as it may take getting used to wearing glasses for the first time. Try masks made of different materials and choose one you find comfortable, making sure it covers your nose and mouth. Sometimes wearing a mask can trigger a dysfunctional breathing pattern in which you unconsciously breathe too quickly through your mouth. If this happens, relax and try breathing in slowly through your nose and keep your mouth closed, then gently breathe out slowly and completely, letting your abdominal muscles relax before starting to breathe in again. Do not use your neck or upper chest muscles to breathe out. Don't focus on your mask and focus instead on your activities. You may take breathing breaks when you are somewhere away from others where it's safe to take off your mask.

Is there any danger from oxygen depletion or carbon dioxide buildup?
No, cloth and surgical masks are permeable, and neither is associated with significant problems involving oxygen or carbon dioxide. Oxygen depletion (hypoxia) cannot occur. There may be a mild increase in carbon dioxide since this is breathed out, but it is at low and safe levels.

What is the most serious outcome associated with wearing a mask?
The most serious harm associated with masks comes from violent confrontations over wearing masks. Mask-wearing has become highly politicized with strong feelings on both sides. Several deaths have occurred in the United States in connection with conflicts over this issue. Some of the misunderstandings

may stem from the difficulty of communicating effectively and establishing personal connections while wearing a mask, since masks hinder our ability to see facial expressions and personally relate to each other. This violence and confrontation points to a need to establish a shared understanding about the purpose of masks and how they benefit everyone.

CHAPTER 8

Workplace Safety

Everyone in the workplace should follow the four-point personal safety strategy, which should also be the cornerstone of every workplace safety policy. Employers have an institutional responsibility to maximize workplace safety by providing the needed resources along with a structure consistent with your personal safety strategy. This chapter offers practical guidance for staying safe in the workplace and providing a workplace that protects everyone in the organization.

What safety measures should my employer provide to keep my workplace safe?
High-risk workplaces prone to infectious clusters tend to be environments where masking is not universal, chances of exposure are higher due to activities such as loud talking and reduced distancing, daily symptom monitoring is not enforced, and regular hand-washing does not occur.

Your employer has an obligation to protect your safety in the workplace, and ideally should provide a structure that supports your personal safety strategy. Below are some workplace measures that support a four-point personal safety strategy:

• Promote regular hand-washing:

- » Clean bathroom facilities regularly and decontaminate surfaces
- » Offer readily accessible, conveniently located hand sanitization
- » Provide reminders to employees to wash hands before eating and entering shared areas
- » Provide disinfectant wipes for work areas
- » Regularly decontaminate high-touch shared areas
- Enforce daily symptom monitoring:
  - » Regularly remind everyone in the organization that daily monitoring is the organization's expectation
  - » Offer paid time-off policies that encourage and support the need for illness leaves of absence
  - » Support and enforce CDC guidelines for staying away from work
  - » Make arrangements to support clinical evaluation and appropriate testing
- Enforce social distancing:
  - » Provide signage and floor/wall markings that support social distancing
  - » Maintain lower building occupancy and use of space
  - » Encourage remote work when possible
  - » Arrange work break and eating areas to support social distancing
- Support universal mask-wearing:
  - » Offer access to high-quality masks
  - » Install Plexiglas protective barriers for extra protection

» Provide face shields to supplement masks
where necessary
» Optimize airflow and ventilation
» Promote and promote flu vaccinations,
since flu and coronavirus are closely related
threats
» Evaluate whether to support coronavirus
vaccinations based on effectiveness and
safety
» Provide wellness and behavioral health
programs that promote safety and well-being

It is important to embed the personal safety strategy into work-place safety so a culture of community safety is maintained.

If I wake up with a mild sore throat, is it okay for me to go to work wearing a mask?
No, you should not go to work and possibly expose others, even if your symptoms are mild and you plan on wearing a mask. Only 30 percent of those infected with coronavirus have a fever at the beginning of their illness, so you should carefully monitor yourself for respiratory symptoms such as a sore throat. Those who are infected with the coronavirus are most infectious in the early stage of infection. If you can work remotely, you may work if you are able, but you should self-isolate.

If I become ill with the coronavirus, how will I know whether I was infected at work if everyone was wearing a mask?
It is often difficult to tell whether an infection is work-related or acquired elsewhere. It is more likely to be work-related if you regularly have face-to-face or close interaction with others at work, although this risk can be substantially reduced

through masking, Plexiglas barriers or face shields, and social distancing. OSHA recommends that employers consider the following factors when deciding whether an infection should be reported to OSHA as work-related:

- An infection is likely to be work-related if any of the following conditions hold:
  - » Several cases develop among workers who work closely together
  - » The infection was contracted shortly after lengthy, close exposure to a particular customer or coworker who has a confirmed coronavirus infection
  - » The infected person has had frequent, close exposure to the general public at work in a locality with ongoing community transmission
- An infection is not likely work related if the infected person has had close and frequent association outside the workplace with someone else who is infected.
- Due weight should also be given to information from medical providers, public health authorities, or the employee.

If you believe that your infection is work-related, it is important to inform your employer since you may be eligible for financial support during your leave of absence as well as for workers' compensation support. Your employer is required to report employee coronavirus infections to OSHA if they are determined to be work-related. In addition, employers may need to meet additional state requirements for reporting.

Can my employer require me to wear a mask?

Yes, your employer may require you to wear a mask. Your employer is required under OSHA law to ensure a safe working environment, and universal mask-wearing may be key to maintaining a safe workplace. Your employer may also require you to follow safety measures including washing hands regularly, daily symptom monitoring, and social distancing. If you have a disability that prevents you from wearing a mask, you may provide this information to your supervisor and request a reasonable accommodation under the Americans with Disabilities Act.

What if I am unable to wear a mask at work because of a medical condition or disability?

You may be eligible for an exemption under the ADA if you have a disability that requires a reasonable accommodation. The CDC indicates several conditions that may make it impossible to wear a mask: difficulty breathing, being incapacitated, and the inability to remove a face mask without assistance. People who are hard of hearing or deaf and those who care for them may also be unable to wear masks if they rely on lipreading to communicate. In this situation, clear masks are a good option.

Possible accommodations for those who can't wear masks include switching to work that allows social distancing, working remotely, or using a clear mask, face shield, or a more wearable mask.

Employers are not required to make accommodations in certain situations, such as those that require a fundamental alteration to the business model, an undue burden, or if the affected individual poses a direct threat to the health or safety of others:

- A fundamental alteration is defined as a modification that would change the nature of the service, program, activity, goods, services, or facilities. It is a change to such a degree that the original program, service, or activity is no longer the same.

- An undue burden is defined as an action that would result in an undue financial or administrative burden. An undue burden is a significant difficulty or expense.
- A direct threat to the health or safety of others is defined as a significant risk to the health or safety of others that cannot be mitigated by a modification of policies, practices, or procedures, or by provision of auxiliary aids or services. The determination that a person poses a direct threat to the health or safety of others may not be based on generalizations or stereotypes about the effects of a particular disability. It must be based on an individual assessment that considers the particular activity and the actual abilities and disabilities of the individual.

These are complicated legal concepts, so you may need to consult your human resources department or seek outside advice from a public agency or legal services if these issues cannot be satisfactorily resolved.

Can my employer require me to be tested for the coronavirus, especially since I am willing to wear a mask?
Yes, the employer may require testing if it is job-related and consistent with business necessity. You may ask your employer about the purpose for the testing to see if it satisfies these criteria. Testing may satisfy these criteria if it is required by the state department of public health for public health reasons or if the testing is necessary to maintain a safe environment for

clients and coworkers. The type of testing may be important, since antibody testing does not provide helpful information for workplace safety purposes.

Does HIPAA prevent me from knowing if someone else whom I work with is infected?
HIPAA (Health Insurance Portability and Accountability Act) generally does not apply to employers. HIPAA only applies to medical providers, hospitals, and other health-care organizations. Still, employers should protect the medical privacy of workers under state privacy laws. Employers are encouraged to notify workers if they have actually been exposed to an infected coworkers or client. Employers should not reveal the identity or provide medical information, but are allowed to inform workers if they have been exposed and should consider being tested or quarantine and monitor for symptoms.

What if I am exposed to an infected person at work while I was wearing a mask?
You should seek medical advice about whether you should be tested or quarantined based on the significance of the exposure. Generally, if you were exposed for 15 minutes or more within six feet of an infected person, you should be quarantined for 14 days and consider being tested. Wearing a mask does not necessarily protect you. The primary purpose of wearing a mask is to reduce the viral spread to others if you are infected.

Is it okay if I take public transportation to commute to work?
If you use public transportation, it is important that you wear a mask and socially distance. A good example of the importance of wearing a mask appears in a published report

about a cluster outbreak in Chongquing, China.[1] A passenger developed a cough before boarding a coach bus with 39 other passengers for a trip lasting over two hours. He did not bring a mask on him and was in a hurry, so he did not wear a face mask in the coach bus. But when he arrived, he bought a mask and wore it on the next leg of his trip, a 50-minute minibus ride with 14 other passengers. A government contact tracing team contacted the passengers on both the coach bus and the minibus after this passenger tested positive. Five people on the coach bus subsequently tested positive within 14 days, while none on the minibus developed symptoms or tested positive.

Is it safer to work remotely?
Many employers have asked employees to work remotely because it keeps building occupancy low and may be a more suitable arrangement during the present state of the pandemic. This issue may need to be individually assessed, taking into account whether you have medical conditions that make you more vulnerable to the disease and whether your employer considers it feasible for you to work remotely. If an employee has a medical condition that amounts to a disability protected by the ADA, he or she should contact Human Resources and seek an accommodation that may possibly allow remote work, although other alternatives may be considered.

How can I stay safe during work breaks and at mealtimes?
Perhaps the most vulnerable periods for exposure occur when people are eating or taking work breaks. When eating, it is critical to maintain social distancing and keep in mind that droplet spread occurs when you are speaking, especially when

---

1   X Liu, S Zhang. Covid-19: face masks and human-to-human transmission. Influenza Other Respiratory Viruses. 2020 Jul; 14(4): 472–473.

people are speaking loudly to each other due to social distancing. Thus, when taking work breaks, it is important to continue wearing your mask and ensure others around you are wearing masks as well.

If I become infected with the coronavirus, when may I return back to work?
You may return back to work under the following conditions:

- Ten days after the first appearance of symptoms and
- Twenty-four hours with no fever without the use of fever-reducing medications and
- Other symptoms are improving.

Most people do not need testing to determine when they can return to work. If your medical provider recommends testing, then they can let you know when you can return to work based on your test results. People who are severely ill may need to stay home longer than 10 days and up to 20 days after symptoms first appear. If you are severely immunocompromised, you may need testing to determine when you can be around others. You will need to discuss this with your medical provider.

CHAPTER 9

The Scientific Basis for Masking: Medical, Biosafety, and Observational Studies

The scientific evidence supporting universal mask-wearing is substantial and advancing rapidly. This chapter describes the evidence found in recent medical research, biosafety testing, and observational studies of households and communities. The next chapter offers an overview of the evidence from population-based studies.

The Characteristics of Coronavirus Transmission

As noted in earlier chapters, the coronavirus infection is primarily transmitted through exhaled small droplets and aerosols. An infected person exhales moisture in the form of small droplets (greater than 5 micrometers) and tiny aerosols (less than 5 micrometers) containing the coronavirus particles. Because masks reduce the quantity of small exhaled droplets containing coronavirus particles, masking has become a common public health strategy to control respiratory infection.

A number of studies on closely related viral infections confirm the effectiveness of masking. Leung and others studied how seasonal coronaviruses, influenza viruses, and rhinoviruses are transmitted in the exhaled breath of those with an acute respiratory illness.[1] While the seasonal coronaviruses are not identical to the coronavirus responsible for this pandemic, they are of the same genus (family), and like their relatives, are transmitted by droplet infection. These studies measured viral RNA found in the respiratory droplets and aerosols exhaled by persons infected with a seasonal coronavirus, influenza virus, or rhinovirus. Viral RNA was found in 30 percent of droplets and 40 percent of aerosols from persons infected with a seasonal coronavirus who were not wearing surgical face masks. However, no seasonal coronavirus was detected in either droplets or aerosols from those wearing masks.

A recent MIT study of respiratory emissions associated with the coronavirus showed that these emissions can take the form of a turbulent gas cloud that can travel up to 23–27 feet, depending on factors such as the person's physiology and the environment's humidity and temperature.[2] This finding underlines the importance of both masks and social distancing in reducing transmission. Another study used a laser-light-scattering methodology to investigate the amount of expelled droplets generated in different contexts. It found that the amount of droplets generated varied with the loudness of speech and increased with coughing.[3] However, when a slightly damp cloth cover was placed over the mouth, the number of droplets was reduced to background level.

---

1   N. H. Leung, D. K. W. Chu, E. Y. C. Shiu, et al. Respiratory virus shedding in exhaled breath and efficacy of face masks. *Nature Medicine* 26:676–680 (2020).

2   L. Bouroulba. Turbulent gas clouds and respiratory pathogen emissions: Potential implications for reducing transmission of Covid-19, *JAMA*, May 12, 2020, 323:1837–1838, May 12, 2020.

3   P. Anfinrud, C. E. Bax, and A. Bax. Visualizing speech-generated oral fluid droplets with laser light scattering. *New England J. Medicine*, 382:20611-2063, May 21, 2020.

The need for universal mask-wearing is driven by clinical evidence that 30 to 40 percent of those infected are asymptomatic or presymptomatic, and symptom-free infected individuals are as infectious as those experiencing symptoms. A study done at a community treatment center in Korea compared the infectivity of 303 symptomatic and 110 asymptomatic infected patients and found that the asymptomatic patients had similar viral concentrations in their upper respiratory tracts to those who were symptomatic.[4] A similar lack of correlation between infectivity and symptoms was found in a study of children. While children are more likely to have mild or no symptoms than adults, children under five years are likely to have higher viral concentrations in their nose and throats than adults, and those ages 5 to 17 have viral concentrations similar to the viral concentrations in adults.[5] Thus, a lack of symptoms or mildness of symptoms does not correlate with reduced infectivity.

These findings point to the need for source control—such as masking—to reduce the amount of droplets and aerosols exhaled by those infected. They also point to the need for universal masking, since almost half of infectious transmission involves infected individuals who do not have symptoms.

The Filtration Capabilities of Masks

Several different biomechanical mechanisms contribute to the ability of masks to filter and reduce the amount of exhaled

4 S. Lee, T. Kim, E. Lee, et al. Clinical course and molecular viral shedding among asymptomatic and symptomatic patients with SARS-CoVid-2 infection in a community treatment center in the Republic of Korea. *Journal of the American Medical Association Internal Medicine*, doi:10.1001/jamainternmed.2020.3862, published online Aug. 6, 2020.

5 T. Heald-Sargent, W. J. Muller, X. Zheng, et al. Age-related differences in nasopharyngeal severe acute respiratory syndrome coronavirus 2 (SARS-CoV-2) levels in patients with mild to moderate coronavirus disease 2019 (COVID-19). *JAMA Pediatrics*, July 30, 2020.doi:10.1001/jamapediatrics.2020.3651.

droplets and aerosols. The dissemination of droplets (greater than 5 micrometers) is affected by environmental factors such as humidity and temperature. Larger droplets tend to settle due to gravity and may be blocked by inertial impaction. The dissemination of aerosols less than 5 micrograms in size is affected by Brownian motion and mechanical interception by filter fibers. Brownian motion is the erratic motion of tiny particles that prevents them from moving in a straight line and increases the likelihood of filtration. Smaller aerosol particles can be stopped and captured by electrostatic attraction, such as from polypropylene fibers. Electrostatic charge is basically static electricity that causes particles to cling to the fibers. Polypropylene has an electrostatic charge and is used primarily in surgical and N-95 respirators. Cotton, with its irregular fiber structure, is better at blocking particles than synthetic materials such as nylon.

The degree of blockage and diffusion depends on the type of mask. The highest level of blockage is provided by N-95 respirators or surgical masks. N-95 respirators are worn by hospital workers who may be exposed to aerosols, especially those working on certain procedures such as bronchoscopy. N-95 respirators fit tightly and should be fitted for size at least annually, and a medical clearance is required to wear them. They filter out 95 percent or more of even the smallest particles (3 microns or less) when exhaled or inhaled. Thus, they also protect the wearer. In hospitals, workers wear them only in patient care areas. N-95 respirators are made of synthetic plastic fibers, including polypropylene.

In contrast, the surgical masks commonly worn in operating rooms provide source control rather than protect the wearer. They also fit more loosely. Hospitals with universal masking have workers in hospitals wear surgical masks unless they are wearing N-95 respirators. Surgical masks may be made of polypropylene.

The cloth masks worn by the public are more loosely fitted than surgical masks. They may be made of cotton or synthetic material. Like surgical masks, their primary purpose is source control and not protection of the wearer.

A Dutch study compared the relative effectiveness of N-95 respirators, surgical masks, and cloth masks (made of tea cloth material). It evaluated adults and children at rest and engaged in different levels of activity. It found that all these masks provided protection by reducing exposure during all types of activities for both adults and children. The N-95 respirator provided the greatest amount of protection. Surgical masks provided about twice as much protection as cloth masks, with adults having more protection than children perhaps because of better-fitting masks. The study concluded that cloth masks also provided a significant degree of protection, although less than the other masks.

An illuminating study by researchers from the University of Illinois at Urbana-Champaign evaluated the ability of a number of common household fabrics to block large, high-velocity droplets.[6] Most fabrics showed a substantial blocking ability with a single-layer blocking efficiency median of 82 percent. Layered fabrics resulted in substantially increased blocking. For example, a mask with two layers of cotton blocked droplets with an efficiency of 94 percent, yet was twice as breathable as a surgical mask.

In another study, Konda and others evaluated various hybrids, such as cotton-silk, cotton-chiffon, and cotton-flannel when multiple layers were used.[7] The filtration efficiency was more than 80 percent for particles less than

---

6   O. Aydin, B. Emon, S. Cheng, et al. Performance of fabrics for home-made masks against the spread of COVID-19 through droplets: A quantitative mechanistic study. *Extreme Mechanics Letters*, vol. 40, Oct. 2020, 100924.

7   A. Konda, A. Prakash, G. A. Moss, et al. Aerosol filtration efficiency of common fabrics used in respiratory cloth masks. ACS Nano, 2020, 14, 5, 6330–6347.

300 nanometers and greater than 90 percent for particles larger than 300 nanometers. The superior performance of hybrid materials may be due to the combined effect of mechanical and electrostatic-based filtration. An important factor affecting the degree of blocking efficiency of a mask is how well it is fitted to the face: Gaps from improper fit can cause a 60 percent decrease in filtration efficiency.

Because these biosafety studies employ varying methodologies and evaluate an array of mask materials in cloth masks, the reported efficiency of filtration varies among them. The major point, however, is that cloth masks can substantially reduce the amount of droplets and aerosols exhaled by the wearer, although in lower proportions than medical masks. It is likely, however, that these studies substantially underestimate the effectiveness of cloth masks for source control. Most of the moisture exhaled is in droplet form, which is effectively blocked by cloth masks. This filtration process thus reduces the transmission rate of the virus.[8]

You have probably heard that wearing a mask is more effective in protecting other people than protecting the wearer. Here's why. If a person without a mask exhales the droplets, these airborne particles rapidly shrink in size from evaporation while in the air. Because the droplets become much smaller once in the air, those particles—now tiny—can make their way through a cloth mask that someone else is wearing. Wearing a mask blocks a higher proportion of the larger droplets that are exhaled by a masked person, stopping the droplets before they evaporate into tiny particles that could penetrate someone else's cloth mask.

It may not be necessary to wear medical respirators with higher filtration rates than those provided by cloth masks. An

8   J. Howard, A. Huang, Z. Li, et al. Face masks against Covid-19: An evidence review. *PNAS*, April 10, 2020, 30(10):1–8.

extensive review of the scientific and medical literature by an international consortium of scientists concluded that if at least 60 percent of people wore masks that are 60 percent effective in blocking viral transmission, similar to the expected performance of a two-layer cotton mask, then the coronavirus pandemic could be stopped.[9]

It should be emphasized that the current scientific evidence has only shown the effectiveness of nonmedical masks for source control. Stately simply, cloth masks protect those near the wearer. Only limited evidence supports the possible protective role of nonmedical masks for wearers themselves. While N-95 respirators are designed to protect the wearer with a filtration efficacy of 95 percent or more, surgical masks may have a filtration efficacy of 75 percent while other, more loosely worn cloth masks may have removal efficiencies in the 30 to 60 percent range.[10] Mask-wearing as part of the four-point safety strategy, including hand-washing and social distancing, however, may offer some protection. For instance, during the SARS pandemic in Hong Kong, those who wore masks frequently in public were about half as likely to be infected as those who did not.[11]

Studies of Households and Communities

Empirical studies of individuals in households and local communities support the conclusion that masks are an effective means of reducing community spread of the coronavirus.

---

9   Note 8.

10 A. Mueller and L. Fernandez. Assessment of fabric masks as alternatives to standard surgical masks in terms of particle filtration efficiency. April 20, 2020.

11 J. T. F. Lau, H. Tsui, M. Lau, and X. Yang. SARS transmission, risk factors, and prevention in Hong Kong. *Emerging Infectious Diseases* 10(4):April 2004. DOI: 10.3201/eid1004.030628.

Households in Beijing

A study of households in Beijing, China, in February and March 2020 evaluated the role of mask-wearing in reducing secondary spread from an infected household member to other household members. This retrospective cohort study identified 335 people in 124 families with at least one laboratory-confirmed coronavirus case in the family. Families with secondary transmission were defined as family members who became infected within two weeks of symptom onset of the primary case. The proportion of family members who subsequently became infected after someone in their household became infected was 23 percent. If all family members were using masks before the initial member became infected, the proportion of those infected after the initial infection dropped by 79 percent. Wearing a mask after the illness onset of the primary case, however, was not found to be significantly protective.

This study thus confirmed that the highest risk of transmission is prior to symptom onset. Viral infectivity is highest two days before symptom onset to the early days of symptoms. The study also showed that hand-washing alone was not effective, but hand-washing combined with mask-wearing showed additional effectiveness in preventing infection.

Case clusters in Hong Kong

A study published in April 2020 evaluated the impact of universal masking in Hong Kong.[12] The government administered a comprehensive testing program for those with respiratory symptoms seen at clinics and hospitals. The government initially required mask-wearing for those with symptoms beginning on December 31, 2019, with China's

---

12 V. C. C. Cheng, S. C. Wong, V. W. M. Chuang, et al. The role of community-wide wearing of face masks for control of coronavirus disease 2019 (COVID-19) epidemic due to SARS-CoV-2. *Journal of Infection* 81 (2020) 107–114.

announcement of a cluster of coronavirus cases. The Hong Kong government reported that soon thereafter, nearly all of its citizens voluntarily wore face masks. To verify this observation, the government conducted surveys of 10,050 people from April 6 to 8, 2020 and found that only 3.4 percent were not wearing masks.

It is not surprising that public adoption of universal masking occurred quickly in Hong Kong. In the SARS coronavirus epidemic, a study of the 1,192 patients with probable severe acute respiratory syndrome demonstrated that frequent mask use in public venues and frequent hand-washing were associated with a decreased risk of transmission. The study researchers concluded that "these practices played an essential role in limiting the spread of the virus in the community in Hong Kong."[13]

In the 2020 study of the coronavirus pandemic, the researchers investigated the effects of masking in Hong Kong by evaluating 14 case clusters of coronavirus infections occurring over the first 100 days of the pandemic. It turned out that all 14 clusters originated in indoor settings.

Of the 961 total cases in the 14 clusters, 112 cases in 11 clusters occurred in association with public activities and settings where masks were not worn, including a restaurant, a bar, and a gym. Only 11 cases in three clusters were associated with workplace settings where masks were worn.

A Meta-Analysis of Observational Data

A meta-analysis is a formal epidemiological study design in which earlier research is investigated so that conclusions can be drawn about a body of research. Because it involves a broad

---

13 J. T. F. Lau, H. Tsui, M. Lau, and X. Yang. SARS transmission, risk factors, and prevention in Hong Kong. *Emerging Infectious Diseases* 10(4):April 2004.

investigation of multiple studies, a meta-analysis may allow a more precise estimate of the effect of an intervention—such as masking—than a single study can. When conducting an empirical analysis of data aggregated from different research studies, researchers must take into consideration variations in the data and determine if their findings can be generalized. Meta-analysis has become a standard means of assessing the research done on a particular issue and has the advantage of not relying on a single study to derive a conclusion.

A systematic review and meta-analysis of the scientific literature on masking was published by Dr. Derek Chu and others for the World Health Organization. It was published in *The Lancet* in June 2020.[14] Among other factors, the systematic review assessed the use of face masks and eye protection to prevent transmission of coronaviruses (including COVID-19, SARS, and MERS). It evaluated 172 observational studies, including 64 COVID-19 studies across 16 countries and 44 relevant comparative studies in healthcare and non-health-care settings that included 25,697 persons. Based on its evaluation and pooling of the data from these studies, the study concluded that face mask use could result in a large reduction in the risk of infection with stronger associations with surgical masks or similar multilayered cotton masks. Eye protection was also associated with less infection. The systematic review concluded, however, that neither masks nor eye protection afforded complete protection. They did not find any striking differences between the effectiveness of face mask use in health-care and community settings. The reviewers observed that masks in general are associated with a large reduction in infection from coronaviruses; however, the

---

14 D. K. Chu, E. A. Aki, S. Duda, et al. Physical distancing, face masks, and eye protection to prevent person-to-person transmission of SARS-CoV-2 and COVID-19: A systematic review and meta-analysis. *The Lancet* 395:10242, 1973–1987, June 27, 2020.

certainty of the effect was not rated as high because the data was based on observational studies, rather than random controlled trials. They concluded that further research, including randomized trials of the effectiveness of different types of masks in the general population and for health-care workers, is needed. However, random controlled trials of masking pose considerable practical and ethical concerns, especially during a global pandemic.

* * *

This chapter has shown that universal mask-wearing is an appropriate response to the biosafety and medical data on the way infectious transmission occurs. The benefits of masking are also supported by observational studies of the transmission of the infection in households and case clusters and by a meta-analysis of data from observational studies. The next chapter describes additional data associated with large populations, including countries and states.

CHAPTER 10

The Case for Masks: Population-Based Studies

Universal masking has been evaluated by experts in the natural and social sciences, epidemiology, and mathematics. A comprehensive evaluation of universal masking includes its real-life impact on populations. This chapter describes examples of population-based empirical studies of US state and international government programs and mathematical modeling of that data. Critics of universal masking, however, point to the lack of randomized controlled trials. I will argue that this limitation should not be the decisive factor in deciding whether masks are effective, given the practical and ethical limitations of randomized trials for masking, especially in light of the current pandemic.

US States

Many states have adopted mandates that require face mask use in public places where social distancing is difficult, such as on public transportation and in retail stores. Other states have mandates that only apply to employees who provide certain services, such as barbers and nail salons. A University of Iowa study evaluated the impact of these two types of state mandates between April 8 and May 15, 2020.[1] The study evaluated the 15 states and the District of Columbia, that had issued government mandates requiring masking in public places, as well as 20 additional states that had the employee-only mandates. The study compared the two groups of states with mandates to the remaining 15 states that did not have state mandates.

The Iowa study found that the daily growth rate of coronavirus infections significantly declined in the states that mandated masks in public places, but not in those states that did not. The daily case rate declined between 0.9 to 2.0 percentage points during each of the four-day intervals following the initiation of the mandate. The decline steadily increased during each of the time intervals.

These declining rates translated to an estimated 230,000 to 450,000 infections prevented by May 22. The states mandating masks only for employees in certain jobs did not show evidence of declines in the rate of infections, perhaps because many businesses had already independently required their employees to wear masks. Thus, there is strong and comprehensive data showing the effectiveness of state mandates for mask-wearing in some public areas.

International

A group of scholars from Yale University compared the impact of the pandemic on countries whose cultural norms support wide-scale masking and those that do not.[2] They found that the average daily growth rate of confirmed positives was 18 percent

1   W. Lyu and G. I. Wehby. Community use of face masks and Covid-19: Evidence from a natural experiment of state mandates in the US. *Health Affairs*, Aug. 2020, 39:8, 1419–1425.

2   J. Abaluck, et al. The case for universal cloth mask adoption and policies to increase supply of medical masks for health workers (Social Science Research Network, Rochester, NY). SSRN Scholarly Paper ID 35678438 (2020).

in countries without preexisting norms for masking, but only 10 percent in countries with such norms. Furthermore, the growth rate of coronavirus deaths was 21 percent in countries without a culture of wide-scale masking, but only 11 percent in countries with such a culture.

An interesting empirical study by Mitze evaluated the impact of a universal mask requirement by the city of Jena and some other regions of Germany.[3] At the beginning of April, Jena was the first city to impose a mandatory masking requirement for those using public transportation and entering retail stores. Six regions adopted similar requirements in April, before universal masking became required throughout Germany at the end of the month. The sequential adoption of the mask requirement created a natural experimental setting that allowed a comparative analysis of the infection rates in Jena and the six regions and other cities and regions that did not adopt the requirement until the end of April.

The research used a synthetic control methodology that compared the two groups of communities only after appropriate adjustments were made based on demographic data to ensure that the synthetic control is properly representative. The demographic considerations included the overall population density, age structure, and health-care system characteristics. Further checks were made on the validity of the data including the absence of early anticipation effects or interference from other events. The synthetic control methodology is widely used to evaluate socioeconomic interventions such as this.

After the face mask requirement was adopted by the city of Jena, there was a reduction of about 25 percent in the

---

3   T. Mitze, R. Kosfeld, J. Rode, and K. Walde. Face masks considerably reduce COVID-19 cases in Germany: A synthetic control method approach. IZA— Institute of Labor Economics, Contract No.: IZA DP No. 13319. Available at: https://ww.iza.org/publications/dp/13319/face-masks-considerably-reduce -covid-19-cases-in-germany-a-synthetic-control-method-approach

cumulative number of reported coronavirus cases after 20 days. The largest reduction, more than 50 percent, was found in the 60-years-and-over age group. The researchers concluded that the mask-wearing policy led to a fall of about 40 percent in the daily growth rate of coronavirus cases. The policy impact was larger for larger cities than for the entire region studied. Overall, the study estimates that the mask requirement resulted in a 40 to 60 percent reduction in the growth rates of infection.

Mathematical Modeling

Mathematical modeling is a critical tool for forecasting the spread of coronavirus. The key concept is based on R0 (pronounced "R naught") that is defined as the average number of people who will become infected from one infected person. R0 is obtained at the start of an epidemic, when everyone is free of the infection and no one has immunity. For example, a R0 of 2.5 means that an infected person will transmit it to an average of 2.5 other people. The coronavirus has a R0 of about 2.4. Later in the epidemic, mathematicians use a different symbol, Re, the effective reproductive number. Re is the number in a population who can be infected by an individual at any specific time. Re changes as the population develops immunity and as people die.

Re is affected by the number of infected people, the number of those susceptible to infection, the contact rate, and the mode of transmission. Human behavior, including masking and social distancing, can also affect Re. If R0 or Re is more than 1.0, the epidemic will increase. However, if R0 or Re is less than 1.0, the epidemic will diminish and end. Re may be used to determine if it is safe for states to reopen. For example, some policy makers consider a Re of 0.7 the standard for reopening. Re may also be used to determine how effective an intervention, such as universal masking, needs to be to diminish and stop an epidemic.

Two of the most widely used models are SEIR (suscep-tible-exposed-infectious-recovered) and ABM (agent-based modeling). The SEIR model assigns people to one of the five categories: susceptible to infection, exposed and not yet infec-tious, infectious, recovered, or dead. Mathematical equations describe the rates at which people move from one category to another, relying on data such as the contact rate, the probabil-ity of transmission, and the duration of the infection.

The ABM type of modeling is a more complex analysis. It simulates the interaction of agents, for example people or groups of people, in order to predict the effects of their behav-ior on the system as a whole. To predict the coronavirus pan-demic spread, an ABM may investigate individual choices on whether and when to wear a mask, as well as the social net-works within which people come into contact.

There are variations of both the SEIR and ABM models as well as other types of modeling. The accuracy of the forecasts made by mathematical modeling depends on the quality of data used by the model and the model's features. Recent mod-eling of the coronavirus pandemic has heavily emphasized the potential importance of universal masking. This emphasis is based on the factors that have been found significant and thus likely to impact the pandemic's development.

Evidence from a SEIR-type model

An international team led by Ngonghala developed a novel SEIR-type mathematical model for assessing the impact of control and mitigation strategies for the coronavirus pan-demic.[4] It is based on US data, particularly from New York, the epicenter of the initial coronavirus wave. It assessed the main intervention strategies including quarantine, isolation,

---

4   C. N. Ngonghala, E. Iboi, S. Eikenberry, et al. Mathematical assessment of the impact of non-pharmaceutical interventions on curtailing the 2019 novel coronavirus. Matt Bioscience, 2020 Jul; 325: 108364.

contact tracing, social distancing, and the use of face masks in public. Based on biosafety data, the study estimated mask-filtering efficacy to range widely, from 20–80 percent for cloth masks to at least 50 percent for well-made, tightly fitting masks made of optimal materials, to 70–90 percent for surgical masks, and over 95 percent typical for N-95 respirators.

The Ngonghala study found that if the masks had a filtering efficacy of 50 percent, the pandemic curve would be greatly flattened. However, the disease would not be entirely eliminated. There would, however, be a significant reduction in the burden of the pandemic. If 75 percent of the NY population wore masks with a 25 percent filtering efficacy, the number of hospitalizations would be reduced by 63 percent. With masks of an efficiency of 75 percent or higher, the pandemic would be eliminated.

Combining strict social distancing (such as that occurring during a state shutdown) with masking increased the effectiveness substantially: Even with masks only moderately effective in filtering (50 percent efficiency), the pandemic would stop. The large effect of masking results from a large proportion of the population wearing masks, even if the masks' filtering efficiency is low. In other words, even wearing a low-quality mask may be acceptable as long as 75 percent or more of the population uses them. The combination of mask-wearing with strict social distancing is a powerful way to stop a pandemic.

Evidence from an ABM-type model

A British team led by Stutt published an analysis based on two models, an ABM model and a SEIR model.[5] They linked the effects of mask-wearing on individual transmission of

---

5   R. O. J. H. Stutt, R. Retkute, M. Bradley, et al. A modelling framework to assess the likely effectiveness of face masks in combination with 'lock-down' in managing the Covid-19 pandemic. *Proceedings of the Royal Society A*, 10 June 2020. https://doi.orgl/10.1098/rspa.2020.0376.

infection with population-level models to assess the effectiveness of mask adoption in different scenarios. They found the most optimal reductions in the Re occur when high-efficacy masks are worn all the time by a high proportion of the population. Similar to the Ngonghala study, the Stutt models demonstrated that if 75 percent of the population wore masks with a filtration efficacy of 75 percent, the pandemic would be halted. However, lower compliance with mask-wearing and masks with lower filtration efficacy may still substantially reduce infection rates.

Mathematical modeling is at the forefront of policy making for the coronavirus pandemic. One of the leading forecasting groups with expertise in modeling the pandemic is the Institute for Health Metrics and Evaluation (IHME) at the University of Washington. Dr. Christopher Murray, the director of IHME, has stated that, "wearing masks can reduce the transmission of the virus by as much as 50 percent, and those who refuse are putting their lives, their families, and their communities at risk."[6]

Randomized Controlled Trials—Why Haven't There Been Any?

Critics of universal masking point to the lack of scientific support from randomized controlled trials. The evaluation of drugs and medical treatments is closely regulated by the Food and Drug Agency, which regularly relies on randomized control trials to compare the outcomes of subjects randomly assigned to a medical intervention to the outcomes for a control group. It is true that there has not been a randomized control trial testing whether cloth masks can protect those

---

6   IHME: New IHME Covid-19 model projects nearly 180,000 US deaths. June 24, 2020.

near an infected wearer.[7] However, there have been limited randomized control trials testing whether medical or cloth masks protect the wearer from other transmissible respiratory viruses.[8] These studies basically show that surgical masks may provide protection against transmissible respiratory viruses, but provide little information about the effectiveness of cloth masks.

Clearly, there are practical and ethical constraints to recruiting participants for trials that would intentionally expose some to the coronavirus. Such exposure would be unethical in light of the dangerous nature of the pandemic. It is also more difficult to study the impact of masking on those who are exposed to the infected person (source control) than to study whether masking protects the wearer. Furthermore, it would not be possible to make such a study "double blind," which would entail concealing the identities of those who are infected or not masked.

Drugs and medical treatments are standardly evaluated by randomized controlled trials due to FDA regulations and financial support from drug companies and NIH research programs. There is no similar structure in place for testing the effectiveness of cloth masks in a standardized way. Standardized testing is further complicated by the fact that many cloth masks are homemade.

---

7   C. R. MacIntyre, H. Seale, T. C. Dung, et al. A cluster randomized trial of cloth masks compared with medical masks in healthcare workers. *BMJ Open* 2015;5:e006577, doi:10.1136/bmjopen-2014-006577; C. R. MacIntyre, A. A. Chughtai, H. Seale, D. E. Dwyer, and W. Quanyi. Human coronavirus data from four clinical trials of masks and respirators. *International Journal of Infectious Diseases* 96 (2020) 631–633.

8   C. R. MacIntyre and A. A. Chughtai. A rapid systematic review of the efficacy of face masks and respirators against coronaviruses and other respiratory transmissible viruses for the community, healthcare workers, and sick patients. *International Journal of Nursing Studies* 108 (2020)103629.

Because masks are part of a public health intervention with broader implications than medical interventions, it makes sense for us to evaluate the full array of interdisciplinary evidence, including biosafety studies and population-based research.

* * *

A growing consensus is emerging in the public health and medical communities that recognizes the importance of masks and accepts the scientific basis for their use.[9] Experts in these areas point to the biosafety, medical, observational, and population-based studies as offering sufficient support.

Critics of masks note that randomized controlled studies are an important way to remove the possibility of confounding factors—the possibility that other factors associated with masks may be the true cause for the reduction in the infection rate described in observational and population-based studies.[10] These types of studies arguably only show correlations.

But when assessing whether the scientific evidence is sufficiently strong to support masks, we need to think about the big picture. There is no medical evidence that finds any significant harm associated with wearing masks,[11] while the coronavirus pandemic represents a substantial danger. Even in the

---

9   T. Greenhalgh, M. B. Schmid, T. Czypionka, D. Bassler, and L. Gruer. Face masks for the public during the covid-19 crisis. *British Medical Journal* 2020; 369:m1435 doi: 10.1136/bmj.m 1435 (9 April 2020); C. M. Clase, E. L. Fu, M. Joseph, et al. Cloth masks may prevent transmission of Covid-19: and evidence-based, risk-based approach. *Annals of Internal Medicine.* https://doi.org/10.7326/M20-2567; Agency for Healthcare Research and Quality. Rapid Evidence Product Version 2.0 (June 24, 2020). Masks for prevention of covid-19 in community and healthcare settings; J. Howard, A. Huang, Z. Li, et al. Face masks against covid-10: an evidence review. *PNAS*, April 10, 2020.

10 T. Jefferson and C. Heneghan. Masking lack of evidence with politics. *CEBM*, July 23, 2020.

11 Agency for Healthcare Research and Quality, supra note 8.

face of scientific uncertainty, we still need to apply the precautionary principle, a long-standing ethical principle of the public health community. The precautionary principle calls on us to deploy scientifically plausible interventions to avoid morally unacceptable harm even if the effectiveness of these interventions is uncertain. In the case of masking, the possible existence of confounding factors is an insufficient reason not to act. Indeed, masks should be always tied to the four-point strategy—washing hands, social distancing, and symptom monitoring along with mask-wearing. If masking reminds people to do things that reduce the risk of infection, this is an acceptable outcome.

CHAPTER 11

Developing a Culture of Community Safety

Your face is the public symbol of your identity. No two faces are identical. You have 43 muscles capable of creating more than 7,000 different expressions, which are intuitively and instantly understood by others and offer the first impression of your character. Your face appears on identification badges because it tells more about you than can be easily communicated in words.

For all these reasons, covering up your face represents a significant loss of an important part of who you are. In light of the immutable link between one's face and one's identity, the outraged response to government masking mandates is understandable—and this means health-care and public safety professionals face an uphill battle in cultivating a culture that not only accepts but also promotes the benefits of universal masking. This chapter explores some of the historical and sociological factors underlying the resistance to masking in the United States and proposes some ways universal masking can be promoted and supported.

Historical Opposition to Masking

Unlike some other countries, US culture lacks a history of universal masking. While there are many photographs of people wearing white masks during the 1918 Spanish flu pandemic, universal masking was not widely embraced, except perhaps in the Midwest and parts of the West Coast, due to strong popular opposition. Experts suggest the controversial public mask requirements failed because they only required masks to be worn outdoors and not when inside public buildings. In addition, masks were neither worn correctly nor consistently.[1]

This popular distrust of masking was reflected in expert opinion of the time. George Soper wrote in *Science* in 1919 about the lessons learned about the Spanish flu pandemic. The second lesson learned was that it was "not desirable to make the general wearing of masks compulsory." (The first, equally counterproductive lesson was that it was "not desirable to close theaters, churches, and schools unless public opinion emphatically demands it.")

The use of surgical masks by doctors and nurses has a separate historical lineage originating with the scientific discovery of the germ theory and the importance of preventing surgical infections. The birth of the surgical mask came from the realization that surgical wounds need protection from the droplets released in the breath of surgeons. By 1933, most surgeons were wearing masks in the operating room.[2] However, regular hospital mask usage never extended much beyond delineated hospital areas, and masks still have not been adopted by the general public in the United States as they have been in Japan, South Korea, and other Asian countries.

---

1   E. T. Ewing. Flu masks failed in 1918, but we need them now. *Health Affairs Blog*, May 12, 2020 DOI: 10.1377/hblog20200508.

2   B. J. Strasser and T. Schlick. The art of medicine: A history of the medical mask and the rise of throwaway culture. *The Lancet* 396, July 4, 2020, 19–20.

Sociological Challenges to Universal Masking

Many of the obstacles to implementing a universal masking policy are rooted in sociological factors. For instance, another reason why universal masking may be difficult to attain is that widespread threats such as pandemics can generate feelings of panic and insecurity, which in turn make people less willing to practice self-sacrifice. In some contexts, a major pandemic can fracture communities and trigger violence and discrimination against stigmatized and scapegoated racial or ethnic groups.[3] In such contexts, it may be difficult to implement a public health initiative that relies on universal behavioral change, especially if the unfamiliar new behavior is intended primarily to benefit others.

Online social networks are another factor that can promote both harmful and beneficial behaviors. For example, in July 2020, a series of false online claims emerged that wearing face masks causes bacterial and fungal pulmonary infections as well as oxygen depletion and carbon dioxide toxicity. While one such post quickly drew more than 5,000 Facebook interactions, what followed was a remarkable series of testimony by nurses, doctors, and other frontline health-care workers who attested to the safety of wearing masks on a daily basis.[4] Major news networks followed this wave of spontaneous clinical testimony by fact-checking and noting the falsity of the claims about health harms associated with masks.

Social media has been found beneficial in other contexts as well. A Dutch study demonstrated the value of a social media campaign that targeted improvements in social distancing and hand-washing to control the coronavirus pandemic.

---

3   J. J. Van Bavel, K. Baiker, P. S. Boggio, et al. Using social and behavioural science to support Covid-19 pandemic response. *Nature Human Behavior* 4, 460–471 (2020).

4   B Dupuy. Posts falsely claim that wearing face masks harms health. AP News, https://apnews.com/afs:Content:9091960069.

The widespread dissemination of this information by news media and social influencers sharing its video and infographics resulted in substantial improvements in these behavioral practices in the Netherlands.[5]

The Psychological Benefits of Masking

A Polish study found that masking offers psychological as well as epidemiological benefits. The researchers evaluated the impact of universal masking on employees returning to the workplace after the pandemic shutdown. They noted the impact of masking in reducing psychological symptoms through reinforcing a sense of personal control, moderating anxiety, and reducing helplessness.[6] A similar study in China reported that universal masking and improvement in workplace hygiene were associated with less severe psychiatric symptoms, particularly from post-traumatic stress.[7]

Building a Culture of Community Safety

It is critical that masking become an accepted part of our culture of community safety because universal masking is essential to successfully stop the pandemic. Everyone needs to wear a mask because it would be impossible to mask only those who

5   H. Yousuf, J. Corbin, G. Sweep, et al. Association of a public health campaign about coronavirus disease 2019 promoted by news media and a social influencer with self-reported personal hygiene and physical distancing in the Netherlands. *JAMA Network Open.* 2020.3(7):e2014323.doi:10.1001/jamanetworkopen.2020.14323.

6   D. Szczesniak, M. Giulkowicz, J. Maciaszek, et al. Psychopathological responses and face mask restrictions during the Covid-19 outbreak: Results from a nationwide survey. *Brain, Behavior, and Immunity* 87 (2020) 1610162.

7   W. Tan, F. Hao, R. S. McIntyre, et al. Is returning to work during the Covid-19 pandemic stressful? A study on immediate mental health status and psychoneuroimmunity prevention measures of the Chinese workforce. *Brain, Behavior, and Immunity* 87 (2020) 84–92.

are infected but asymptomatic. Universal masking also reduces the possible stigmatization of those wearing masks, such as members of some minority groups and those who are sick.

The announcement by the CDC on July 14, 2020, of its commitment to universal masking was a call to the scientific and public health communities to clearly communicate why universal masking is necessary. Local community leaders should also take the lead in establishing a culture of community safety that supports universal masking and other safety measures. This includes support by employers for universal masking in workplaces.

Organizations can play a role by developing structures that promote collaborative relationships between workers and managers to promote workplace safety. This has been the standard practice in hospitals, which cultivate their culture of safety by relying on workplace safety committees to bring together representatives from nursing, physician groups, safety officers, occupational health, buildings and grounds management, and other departments. At the Brigham and Women's Hospital, this safety group is called the Environment of Care committee. It reviews data and listens to frontline workers about their environmental safety concerns and work-related injuries or illnesses. This committee is the hospital's primary means of developing a community understanding about workplace safety risk and how to support interventions based on regularly collected data.

While a pandemic can fracture a community, it can also contribute to a sense of shared identity. People sharing an experience may empathize with each other and display remarkable altruism in supporting each other. Stronger scientific communication may foster a consensus about the need for universal masking. We have a common identity in facing the same risk and a shared fate. And we need to effectively communicate that universal masking means "You are protecting me, and I am protecting you."

CHAPTER 12

Masks: The Most Important Public Health Tool

The scientific support for masking is strong, convincing, and growing rapidly. Universal mask wearing can become our most important public health tool in the battle against the coronavirus if we can make it an emblem of our personal safety strategy. It is especially critical because the virus can be spread by those who are not symptomatic, making it particularly contagious.

Observational studies show that consistent masking in a variety of situations and places reduces the infection rate among those who are exposed to infected people. A meta-analysis of the accumulated data from these observational studies confirms the significant impact of masking. Most importantly, the recent adoption of state and national masking mandates shows that they result in a substantial reduction in infection rates and deaths from coronavirus. The data that we have gathered through this empirical research has been used in mathematical modeling to provide important forecasting of the spread of the virus.

Given these facts, a few key questions remain: First, how can we finally end the pandemic, and what role can masking play in this effort? Second, given the benefits of masking, what can we do as a society to better promote it?

Achieving Herd Immunity: Is It Possible?

The ultimate goal of our efforts, of course, is to end the coronavirus pandemic for good. Several types of interventions can potentially reduce the effective reproductive number, Re, to below 1.0, the level at which the pandemic will diminish and end. Some of these include developing medicines that are highly effective in promoting recovery or in preventing infections from occurring, increasing the number of those who become naturally immune after becoming infected, vaccinating a sufficient number of people with an effective vaccine, or universal masking. Unfortunately, the development of highly effective medications or those capable of preventing infection seems unlikely in the near future and may take many years to accomplish, if even possible.

The possibility of keeping the Re below 1.0 through the development of natural immunity or by vaccination entails achieving what is called herd immunity. Herd immunity refers to the idea that if a sufficient number of people in a community become immune to the virus, it can no longer spread because there is no longer a sufficient number of susceptible people. While we do not yet know the precise percentage of immunity required to attain herd immunity from the coronavirus, it is generally estimated that 65 to 75 percent of the population may need to develop immunity for herd immunity to take effect. (In contrast, the percentage required for herd immunity to the flu is known to be about 60 to 70 percent, since it is less infectious than the coronavirus and has a R0 equal to 1.3.)

The only country that has attempted to achieve herd immunity by not controlling the spread of infections is Sweden. While it is too early to judge the Swedish approach, its death rate from coronavirus is 5 to 10 times higher than that of neighboring countries, and the immunity level of its population based on antibody testing is less than 10 percent.

If the United States similarly relied on achieving herd immunity through natural spread, it is estimated that about 1 to 2 million people would die before it could be achieved. In addition, hospitals and medical providers are likely to be overwhelmed by the large number of patients if there is no attempt by government to control the spread of the virus.

Many have pinned their hopes on achieving herd immunity through vaccination. While development of an effective vaccine is possible, it is far from certain. An excellent coronavirus vaccine is likely to be 70–75 percent effective, with the minimum effectiveness for FDA approval defined as 50 percent. (The average flu vaccine is 60 percent effective for one season.) The length of immunity following vaccination is also unknown, especially given the short persistence of antibodies (they persist for just a few months after natural infection). Furthermore, because of infrastructure limitations, it will take time to produce sufficient quantities of the vaccine and vaccinate all who wish to be vaccinated, and a slow ramp-up is expected. Most of the potential vaccines require cold storage at temperatures as low as minus 80 degrees Celsius, and many must be given in two doses delivered a month apart. While the development of the vaccines has been supported by the federal government's Operation Warp Speed, there is public concern about the uncertainty of unforeseen side effects: Polls have shown that about 20–30 percent of Americans have already indicated they will not take the vaccine.

In short, we cannot rely on vaccination alone as the silver bullet for ending the pandemic. The approach most likely to be successful is using universal masking as the primary means of protecting the population, while simultaneously vaccinating as many people as possible. Universal mask-wearing replicates the effects of herd immunity by decreasing the rate of infective spread. The percentage of the population, perhaps 80–90 percent, likely to wear masks in public spaces is higher than the percentage likely to become immune by vaccination, which would be 45 percent if the vaccine is 75 percent effective with 60 percent of the population participating.

Thus, the combination of universal mask wearing and vaccination may result in the successful management and control of the pandemic spread. Iboi and others have employed mathematical modeling to evaluate the relationship between these two approaches.[1] For a vaccine with a protective efficacy of 80 percent, at least 82 percent of the population needs to be vaccinated to achieve herd immunity. However, the prospect of obtaining herd immunity is greatly enhanced if vaccination is combined with a universal masking program that includes social distancing. For example, if 100 percent of the population wears masks, herd immunity can occur with a vaccination coverage of only 46 percent. Alternatively, if mask compliance is only 50 percent, then 72 percent of the population needs to be vaccinated. Assuming this model, a more realistic way to reach herd immunity would be to have 50 to 60 percent of the population vaccinated and universal masking compliance at 85 to 95 percent.

The reason masks are the most important public health tool is that we currently know more about the efficacy of universal masking (as part of the four-point strategy that also includes washing hands, social distancing, and daily symptom monitoring) than about other possible interventions. Furthermore, while the efficacy and the side effects of vaccination are currently unknown, source control is a public health intervention well understood in occupational and environmental medicine, as well as in infection control. Often, the best opportunity to prevent harm is in directly controlling the source of the undesired exposure. We have in

---

1   E. A. Iboi, C. N. Ngonghala, and A. B. Gumel. Will an imperfect vaccine curtail the Covid-19 pandemic in the U.S.? *Infectious Disease Modelling* 5 (2020) 510–524.

our grasp the ability to control the pandemic, especially if we can improve the quality of masks and public participation in universal mask wearing. As an added benefit, universal masking allows us to avoid reverting to government lockdowns. In short, when practiced consistently along with social distancing, universal masking allows more freedom of activity than stay-at-home orders.

The Economic and Practical Case for Promoting Masks

Given the central role of masks in the current public health emergency, it is astonishing that we are relying on people to obtain their own masks with little attempt to standardize the efficacy of mask filtration or to subsidize research into improving the breathability and fit of masks. While it is critical for the federal government to invest billions of dollars in developing vaccinations, we have failed to invest significant resources in a universal mask program, despite its similarly high potential value.

A Goldman Sachs research group evaluated three data sources to quantify the value of masks in the economic recovery after the first pandemic wave: (1) a US regional data panel that related infection rates and fatalities to the introduction of state mandates; (2) a large international country-level cross-section of data correlating cumulative infection and fatalities to the lag between the onset of spread and the introduction of mask mandates by country; and (3) a smaller international country-level study that found a correlation between infection rates and fatalities and lags in mask usage.

Not surprisingly, the Goldman Sachs research group found that in June 2020, mask-wearing was associated with significantly better outcomes.[2] They reached this conclusion

---

2   J. Hatzius, D. Struyven, and I. Rosenberg. Goldman Sachs Research. Face Masks and GDP, 29 June 2020.

after analyzing each of three data sets and determined that it reflected the largely causal impact of masks rather than a correlation with other factors, such as reduced mobility or avoidance of large gatherings. Goldman Sachs estimated that a national mask mandate would increase the percentage of people wearing masks by 15 percent and replace the need for state lockdowns that would otherwise reduce the US GDP by nearly 5 percent, a projected savings of $1 trillion.

With so much at stake, in terms of lives and finance, we need to support and promote universal masking by encouraging the production of masks with high filtration efficacy, comfortable fit, and breathability. This will require giving the Food and Drug Agency new authority to develop standards to evaluate mask efficacy. The National Institutes of Health should prioritize the funding of research aimed at evaluating and improving masks used by the public. It is important to quickly evaluate face shields, clear masks, and materials that may be used to manufacture better masks. We should make masks freely available to encourage public use, as some municipalities and states have begun to do, especially for passengers entering public transportation.

Federal and State Mandates and Best Practices for Enforcing Them

Thirty-three states have adopted mandates requiring masks in public areas. Most states have imposed fines for enforcement. A few counties have imposed short jail sentences and fines. There is no current federal mandate in the United States, although universal masking is recommended by the CDC. In this context, mandatory rules would be helpful not so much for enforcement purposes, but rather to reinforce social support for our cultural commitment to a public health principle. This is why the Mass General Brigham hospital system has a mandatory flu vaccination program for all employees, whether or not they work at a hospital site. It is a condition of employment, with a formal exemption process for medical and religious reasons. Less than two percent of employees obtain exemptions, and only a handful have decided to leave their jobs because of it. A universal flu vaccination program for a hospital is a commitment to caring for patients, protecting the health-care workforce, and highlighting the importance of public health in communities.

As a practical matter, however, it is impossible to strictly enforce universal masking in all public areas. We will not achieve 90 to 95 percent compliance through heavy-handed enforcement of fines or arresting people. Indeed, there is the danger of uneven enforcement, especially in minority neighborhoods, and deaths have occurred in connection with violent disagreements about the need for mask wearing. Instead, police should be handing out masks rather than writing tickets or imposing fines. Public health has been most effective in promoting behavioral change through empathy and education, not through shame. We should engage in sincere and respectful conversation, knowing that science and public health are on our side. And we need to make sure quality masks are ubiquitous and universally accessible.

* * *

This pandemic has taken its toll on all of us. We have all experienced loss and suffered from self-isolation. Asking people to wear masks is asking for additional self-sacrifice and altruism at a time when life has already been difficult and unfair. Although safe, masks can be uncomfortable, make it more difficult to breathe freely, and are a nuisance to keep putting on. Moreover, masks are reminders that the pandemic is still with us. We must empathize with those who don't wish to

wear masks. We should respond to their concerns by finding ways to make masks more effective, comfortable, and
accessible. Somehow, we might even find a way to celebrate
masks, as they may be our best hope for a different and better
tomorrow. As the lyrics of the Skagit Valley Chorale's opening
rehearsal song tell us, we must find a way to sing on.

APPENDIX A

Scientific Research and Medical References

This appendix contains a selected bibliography of scientific research and medical articles with descriptive summaries. For the most up-to-date information about specific issues, it is important to check with CDC recommendations because of the evolving scientific information. The CDC has an extensive web site with detailed information. Medical providers and public health experts rely on CDC recommendations when they make medical and public health decisions.

Abaluck J, Chevalier J, Christakis NA, et al. The case for universal cloth mask adoption & policies to increase the supply of medical masks for health workers, April 1, 2020 (white paper by interdisciplinary group at Yale University that supports universal masking of public with cloth masks).

Agency for Healthcare Research and Quality. Masks for prevention of Covid-19 in community and healthcare settings. Rapid Evidence Product Version 2.0 (June 24, 2020) (describing evidence-based review on facemasks including cloth masks in preventing coronavirus infection).

American Academy of Dermatology Association. 9 ways to prevent face-mask skin problems. https://www.aad.org/

public/everyday-care/skin-care-secrets/face/prevent-face
-mask-skin-problems (offering advice on skin care when
wearing masks).

Aydin O, Emon B, Cheng S, et al. Performance of fabrics for
home-made masks against the spread of Covid-19 through
droplets: A quantitative mechanistic study. Extreme
Mechanics Letters, Volume 40, Oct. 2020, 100924 (mea-
suring filtration efficacy of cloth masks).

Bourouiba L. Turbulent gas clouds and respiratory pathogen
emissions: Potential implications for reducing transmission
of Covid-19. Journal of the American Medical Association,
May 12, 2020, 323 (18): 1837–1838 (researching gas cloud
of droplets from a human sneeze).

Brooks JT, Butler JC, Redfield RR. Universal masking to prevent
SARS-CoV-2 transmission—The time is now. Journal of the
American Medical Association, July 14, 2020;324(7):635–
637. doi:10.1001/jama.2020.13107 (announcing CDC
support for universal masking of the public).

Cheng VCC, Wong SC, Chuang VWM, et al. The role of
community-wide wearing of face mask for control of coronavirus disease 2019 (Covid-19) epidemic due to SARS-
CoV-2. Journal of Infection 81 (2020) 107–114 (providing
data from Hong Kong of infected cases of clusters in relationship to activities without masking).

Chu DK, Aki EA, Duda S, et al. Physical distancing, face
masks, and eye protection to prevent person-to-person
transmission of SARS-CoV-2 and Covid-19: A systematic
review and meta-analysis. The Lancet, Vol. 395 (10242),
1973–1987, June 27, 2020 (providing a systematic review
and meta-analysis to assess the use face masks and other
prevention measures to prevent transmission of the pandemic coronavirus and other types of coronaviruses).

Clase CM, Fu EL, Joseph M, et al. Cloth masks may prevent
transmission of Covid-19: An Evidence-based, risk-based

approach. Annals of Internal Medicine, https://doi.
org/10.7326/M20-2567, May 22, 2020 (describing review
of evidence).

Draazen JM, Harrington DP, McMurray JJV, Ware JH, Woo J.
Evidence for health decision making – Beyond randomized,
controlled trials. The New England Journal of Medicine,
2017; 377:465–475, DOI:101056/NEJMra1614394
(describing limits to reliance on randomized controlled
trials).

Edelstein P, Ramakrishnan L. Report on facemasks for the
general public – An update. 07 July 2020, Royal Society
DELVE Initiative (providing review of empirical evidence).

Frieden TR. Evidence for health decision making – Beyond
randomized, controlled trials. The New England Journal
of Medicine 2017; 377:465–475, DOI: 10.1056/
NEJMra1614394 (describing limitations to reliance on
randomized controlled trials).

Gandhi M, Beyrer C, Goosby E. Masks do more than protect others during Covid-19: Reducing the inoculum of
SARS-CoV-2 to protect the wearer. Journal of General
Internal Medicine 2020 https://doi.org/10.1007/s11606-
020-06067-8 (describing theory that masks may provide
protection to wearer by reducing dose of infection).

Greenhalgh T, Schmid MB, Czypionka T, et al. Face masks
for the public during the covid-19 crisis. British Medical
Journal 2020; 369:m1435 doi: 10.1136/bmj.m1435 (published 9 April 2020) (describing review of scientific evidence and reliance on precautionary principle).

Hamner L, Dubbel P, Capron I, et al. High SARS-CoV-2
attack rate following exposure at a choir practice – Skagit
county, Washington, March 2020. MMWR, May 15,
2020, 69 (19):606–610 (describing coronavirus cluster
among choir after two rehearsals).

Heald-Sargent T, Muller WJ, Zheng X, et al. Age-related differences in nasopharyngeal severe acute respiratory syndrome coronavirus 2 (SARS-CoV-2) levels in patients with mild to moderate coronavirus disease 2019 (Covid-19). JAMA Pediatrics, published online July 30, 2020 (finding that children under 5 years with mild to moderate coronavirus infection have higher amounts of virus in their nose and throat compared to older children and adults).

Hendrix MJ, Walde C, Findley K, Trotman R. Absence of apparent transmission of SARS-CoV-2 from two stylists after exposure at a hair salon with a universal face covering policy—Springfield, Missouri, May 2020. MMWR, Jul. 17, 2020, 69 (28): 930–932 (describing the lack of transmission by 2 masked hair stylists infected with coronavirus to their 139 masked clients).

Howard J, Huang A, Li Z, et al. Face masks against Covid-19: An evidence review. Proceedings of the National Academy of Sciences of the USA, April 10, 2020. (providing medical literature review and policy recommendations).

Iboi EA, Ngonghala, Gumel AB. Will an imperfect vaccine curtail the Covid-19 pandemic in the U.S.? Infectious Disease Modeling 5 (2020) 510–524. (mathematical modeling the combination of universal mask wearing and vaccination on infection rates).

Jefferson T, Jones M, Ansari LAA, et al. Physical interventions to interrupt or reduce the spread of respiratory viruses. Part I—face masks, eye protection and person distancing; systematic review and meta-analysis. (pre-print) https://www.medrxiv.org/content/10.1101/2020.03.30.20047217v2 (updating a Cochrane review that included a meta-analysis of observational studies during the SARS outbreak of 2003).

Kissler SM, Tedijanto C, Goldstein E, et al. Projecting the transmission dynamics of SARS-CoV-2 through the postpandemic period. Science 368, 860–868 (2020), 1–9 (describing several alternative models of the remainder of the pandemic activity).

Klompas M, Morris CA, Sinclair J, Pearson M, Shenoy ES. Universal masking in hospitals in the Covid-19 era. The New England Journal of Medicine 2020; 382:e63 DOI: 101056/NEJM p2006372 (describing state of universal masking in hospitals).

Konda A, Prakash A, Moss GA, et al. Aerosol filtration efficiency of common fabrics used in respiratory cloth masks. ACS Nano 2020, 14, 5, 6339–6347 (evaluating filtration efficiencies for various fabrics).

Konda A, Prakash A, Moss GA, et al. Visualizing speech-generated oral fluid droplets with laser light scattering. New England Journal of Medicine, 2020; 382:2061–2063 (describing scattering of droplets that is emitted by speaking).

Lau JTF, Tsui H, Lau M, Yang X. SARS transmission, risk factors, and prevention in Hong Kong. Emergency Infectious Disease 10(4):587–592 (describing that frequent mask use in public venues was a protective factor in SARS epidemic).

Lee B, Raszka WV. Covid-19 transmission and children: The child is not to blame. Pediatrics 146(2), August 2020:e2020004879 (providing summary of data concerning transmission by children).

Lee, S, Kim T, Lee E, et al. Clinical course and molecular viral shedding among asymptomatic and symptomatic patients with SARS-CoV-2 infection in a community treatment center in the Republic of Korea. JAMA Internal Medicine, published online Aug. 6, 2020. Doi:10.1001/jamaint ernmed.2020.3862 (describing that asymptomatic patients had similar amounts of virus concentration in respiratory tract compared to symptomatic patients).

Liu X, Zhang S. Covid-19: Face masks and human-to-human transmission. Influenza and Other Respiratory Viruses. 2020 Jul.; 14(4): 472–473 (describing cluster of cases associated with an infected person using public transportation).

Loch M, Dafoe N, Mahony J, et al. Surgical mask vs N95 respirator for preventing influenza among health care workers: A randomized trial. Journal of the American Medical Association, Nov. 4, 2009, 302(17):1865–1871 (concluding that use of surgical masks by nurses in hospitals resulted in similar rates of flu infection compared to those who wore N95 respirators).

Mulder R, Singh A, Hamilton A, et al. The limitations of using randomized controlled trials as a basis for developing treatment guidelines. Evidence-Based Mental Health. 2018 Feb. 21(1):4–6 (describing limitations of randomized controlled trials as an evidentiary requirement).

Neupane BB, Mainali S, Sharma A, Giri B. Optical microscopic study of surface morphology and filtering efficiency of face masks. Peer Journal, vol. 7, 2019, 7e7142. PMC6599448 (describing filtering efficiencies of cloth face masks).

Ngonghala CN, Iboi E, Eikenberry S, et al. Mathematical assessment of the impact of non-pharmaceutical interventions on curtailing the 2019 novel coronavirus. Math Bioscience 2020 Jul; 325: 108364 (mathematical modeling of impact of masking on pandemic).

Smith JD, MacDougall CC, Johnstone J, et al. Effectiveness of N95 respirators versus surgical masks in protecting health care workers from acute respiratory infection: a systematic review and meta-analysis. Canadian Medical Association Journal, May 17, 2016, 188(8), 567–574 (providing meta-analysis showing that it is not definitive that N95 respirators are superior to surgical masks in protecting health care workers against transmissible acute respiratory infections in clinical settings).

Stutt ROJH, Gilligan CA, Colvin J. A modelling framework to assess the likely effectiveness of facemasks in combination with 'lock-down' in managing the Covid-19 pandemic. Proceedings of the Royal Society, June 2020, 476:2238, (describing two mathematical models that show face masks use by public could make major contribution to reducing the impact of the pandemic).

Szczesniak D, Ciulkowicz M, Maciaszek J, et al. Psychopathological responses and face mask restrictions during the Covid-19 outbreak: Results from a nationwide survey. Brain, Behavior, and Immunity 87 (2020) 161–162 (describing reduction in psychiatric symptoms by universal mask wearing at work when reopening after pandemic in Poland).

Tan W, Hao F, McIntyre RS, et al. Is returning to work during the Covid-19 pandemic stressful? A study on immediate mental health status and psychoneuroimmunity prevention measures of Chinese workforce. Brain, Behavior, and Immunity 87 (2020) 84–92 (describing how hand hygiene and wearing face masks were associated with a lower prevalence of psychiatric symptoms for workers returning to work during reopening in China).

Verma S, Dhanak M, Frankenfield J. Visualizing the effectiveness of face masks in obstructing respiratory jets. Phys. Fluids 32, 061708 (2020); doi: 10.1063/5.0016018 (describing experiment that visualized droplet stream associated with coughs and sneezes).

Victora CG, Habicht, JP, Bryce J. Evidence-based public health: Moving beyond randomized trials. American Journal of Public Health, March 20004, 94(3);400–405 (distinguishing between medical interventions needing randomized controlled trials for evaluation as compared to public health interventions that do not require).

Wang X, Pan Z, Cheng Z. Association between 2019 CoV transmission and N95 respirator use. Journal Hospital Infect. 2020 May; 105(1): 104–105 (comparing infection rate among those wearing N-95 respirators with those not masked).

Wang X, Ferro EG, Zhou G, et al. Association between universal masking in a health care system and SARS-CoV-2 positivity among health care workers. JAMA, 2020, 324(7);703–704 (describing decrease in test positivity rate after universal masking adopted by hospital system).

Wang Y, Tian H, Zhang L, et al. Reduction of secondary transmission of SARS-CoV-2 in households by face mask use, disinfection and social distancing: a cohort study in Beijing, China. BMJ Global Health 2020;5:e002794 (describing transmission within households and impact of mask use).

Zhang L, Peres TG, Silva MV, Camargos P. What we know so far about coronavirus disease 2019 in children: A meta-analysis of 551 laboratory-confirmed cases. Pediatric Pulmonology 2020; 1–13 (describing epidemiology of infections among children).

APPENDIX B

Policy and Law References

This appendix provides a selected bibliography of articles that describe the historical, sociological, empirical policy analysis, and legal perspectives.

History

Ewing ET. Flu masks failed in 1918, but we need them now. Health Affairs Blog, https://www.healthaffairs.org/do/10.1377/hblog20200508.769108/full/ (describing mask use by public in 1918 flu pandemic)

Soper GA. The lessons of the pandemic. Science 49, 501–506 (1919) (describing lessons learned from 1918 flu pandemic)

Strasser BJ, Schlich T. The art of medicine: A history of the medical mask and the rise of throwaway culture. The Lancet, 396:19–20, July 4, 2020 (describing history of surgical mask use).

Sociology

Synnott A. Truth and goodness, mirrors and masks – Part I: A sociology of beauty and the face. The British Journal of Sociology, 40(4) (Dec. 1989), 607–636 (describing social significance of beauty and the face).

Van Bavel JJ, Baicker K, Boggio PS, et al. Using social and behavioural science to support Covid-19 pandemic response. Nature Human Behaviour 4, 460–471 (2020) (describing a number of sociological issues related to the coronavirus pandemic).

Social, Economic, and Policy Empirical Research

Chernozhukov V, Kasahara H, Schrimpf P. Causal impact of masks, policies, behavior on early Covid-19 pandemic in the U.S. The Institute for Fiscal Studies, DOI 10.1920/wp.cem.2020.2420 (describing impact of various policies adopted by US states on the spread of the pandemic).

Hatzius J, Struyven D, Rosenberg I. *Face masks and GDP*, Goldman Sachs Research. June 29, 2020. https://www.golmansachs.com/insights/pages/face-masks-and-gdp.html (describing analysis of three sets of data relevant to public masking and the coronavirus pandemic and providing an economic analysis).

Lyu W, Wehby GL. Community use of face masks and Covid-19: Evidence from a natural experiment of state mandates in the US. Health Affairs 39, No. 8 (2020) 1419–1425 (analyzing data of the impact of state mandates requiring masking by the public on the growth rate of the coronavirus).

Mitze T, Kosfeld R, Rode J, Walde K. Face masks considerably reduce Covid-19 cases in Germany: A synthetic control method approach. IZA Institute of Labor Economics, June 2020, IZA DP No.1 13319, 1–29 (describing the relationship between mandatory masking requirements by German regions with pandemic infection rates).

Yousuf H, Corbin J, Sweep G, et al. Association of a public health campaign about coronavirus disease 2019 promoted by news media and a social influencer with self-reported personal hygiene and physical distancing in the

Netherlands. Journal of the American Medical Association Network Open, 2020.3(7):e2014323.doi:10.1001/jamanetworkopen.2020.14323 (describing successful impact of a media campaign to improve personal hygiene and physical distancing).

Zhang L, Shen M, Ma X, et al. What is required to prevent a second major outbreak of SARS-CoV-2 upon lifting quarantine in Wuhan City, China. The Innovation, 2020 May 21; 1(1): 100006 (describing the need to have a high mask usage to prevent second wave in Wuhan, China).

Law and Policy

Cordaro TL. Navigating employer obligations to provide employees with masks, face coverings. The National Law Review, Sept. 13, 2020, X(257) (describing employer obligations).

Disability Rights California and Disability Education and Defense Fund. Covid-19: Face masks and people with disabilities. https://www.disabilityrightsca.org/post/covid-19-face-masks-and-people-with-disabilities (nonprofit advocacy group's recommendations regarding mask policies and ADA).

Atul Gawande. Amid the Coronavirus crisis, A regimen for reentry, The New Yorker, May 13, 2020 (describing hospital mask and safety initiatives and possible way to re-open the country).

Gatter R, Mohapatra S. COVID-19 and the Conundrum of Mask Requirements, 77 Washington & Lee Law Review Online 17 (2020), https://scholarlycommons.law.wlu.edu/wlulr-online/vol77/iss1/2m (cautioning against mask mandates because of potential for discrimination).

Minnesota Department of Health. Best practices for masks: Considerations for people with disabilities and special health needs. https://www.health.state.mn.us/diseases/ coronavirus/guidemasks.pdf (state agency recommendations for enforcing mask practices and considerations for people with disabilities).

National Safety Council. *Safer: Safe actions for employee returns.* Version 2, Release date: 6/8/20. https://www.nsc.org/Portals/0/Documents/NSC Documents_Advocacy/Safety%20at%20Work/covid-19 /SAFER%20Framework%20Summary050620 .pdf?ver=2020-05-06-162456-463 (recommendations for safe operations for employers and workers in response to the pandemic).

Northwest ADA Center. Face coverings and businesses: Balancing the ADA with public health during Covid-19. http://nwadacenter.org/factsheet/face-coverings-and -businesses-balancing-ada-public-health-during-covid-1 9–0 (nonprofit advocacy group's recommendations with regards to masks and accommodation requirements).

Pendo E, Gatter R, Mohapatra S. Resolving tensions between disability rights law and Covid-19 mask policies. Saint Louis University School of Law, Summer 2020. https:// scholarship.law.slu.edu/faculty (analyzing the application of disability rights law to mask policies).

Southeast ADA Center and Burton Blatt Institute at Syracuse University. The ADA and Face Mask Policies. Updated: 8/20/2020. https://www.adasoutheast.org/ada/publica- tions/legal/ada-and-face-mask-policies.php#t3a (nonprofit advocacy group's recommendations regarding the ADA and mask policies)

U.S. Department of Health and Human Services, Centers for Disease Control and Prevention. CDC activities and initiatives supporting Covid-19 response and the presi- dent's plan for opening America up again. May 2020 https:

//stacks.cdc.gov/view/cdc/88478 (describing the phases of reopening states after the first wave).

U.S. Department of Labor, OSHA. Guidance on preparing workplaces for Covid-19. OSHA 3990-03 2020 https://www.osha.gov/Publications/OSHA3990.pdf (federal gov ernment recommendations for workplace safety).

U.S. Department of Labor, Wage and Hour Division. Families First Coronavirus Response Act: Employer paid leave requirements. https;//www.dol.gov/agencies/whd/pandemic/ffcra-employer-paid-leave (employer paid leave requirements that require paid sick leave or expanded family medical leave for reasons related to the pandemic).

U.S. Equal Employment Opportunity Commission. Pandemic preparedness in the workplace and the Americans with Disabilities Act. https://www.eeoc.gov/laws/guidance/pandemic-preparedness-workplace-and-americans-disabilities-act#secB (pandemic preparedness issues and the ADA).

Acknowledgments

I am deeply grateful for the opportunity to serve the employees and others who work at the Massachusetts General Hospital, Brigham and Women's Hospital, and the Mass General Brigham system. I will always admire their courageous dedication to providing outstanding patient care during this dangerous pandemic. I value my collaborations with those in the Workplace Health and Wellness division and the support for workplace health from hospital leadership including the Mass General Brigham chief clinical officer, Dr. Gregg Meyer, and chief human resource officer, Rose Sheehan. I thank Boston College for the opportunity to teach health law and policy and am greatly appreciative of encouragement from my colleagues, including Mary Sarah Bilder, Fred Yen, Dan Coquillette, Diane Ring, and the law school dean, Vincent Rougeau. I could not have written this book without the capable assistance of Taylor Vitelli, careful editing by Felicia Lee, and thoughtful guidance from the publisher, especially from Abigail Gehring and Tad Crawford. I dedicate this book to my parents, Doris and Ben Hashimoto, and to my family, Vicky, Gary, and Sachi.

Index

A

accommodations at
  employment for a
  disability, 61–62, 64
adverse effects
  breathable, 55
  carbon dioxide build up,
    55, 89
  infectious spread, 29
  medical reasons not to
    wear, 53–54
  oxygen depletion, 55, 89
  skin problems, 54–55
  violent confrontation,
    55–56
aerosolization, 13
airflights, 43
asymptomatic transmission,
  11, 14–15, 20, 30, 49, 68,
  90–91

B

bars, 20–21, 29, 40, 74

beards, 34
biosafety studies, 66, 71, 76,
  82, 85
business responsibilities
  additional, 57–65
  mask policy, 61

C

carbon dioxide, 53, 55, 89
CDC
  hospital guidelines, 31
  reversal of mask wearing
    policy, 10
  universal mask use, 10–11
children
  under age 2 years, 50
  choosing mask, 51–52
  clear masks, 50
  face shields, 50
  mask wearing, 49–52
  masks at school, 50
  summer camps, 52

teaching to wear, 51
when should not wear
mask, 50
China, Beijing, 73
clear masks
children, 50
description, 31–32, 35
communication with public,
91
company policy, mask
requirement, 61
contact tracing, 6, 44, 64, 82
culture of community safety,
23–29, 59, 87–91

D
daily symptom check *see*
symptom check
disability, accommodations
for, 61–62, 64
droplet transmission, 3, 12–
15, 17, 20, 31–32, 35–38,
44, 47, 64, 66–71

E
ear irritation, 54–55
economic savings, 96–97
employee health services, 8,
26–28
employer responsibilities,
57–58, 60–64, 91
exhalation valve, 37

exposures
air flights, 43
bars, 20–21
eating, 64–65
hair salon and barber shop,
5–6
high risk situations, 20–21
hotel, 42–43
restaurants, 21
significant exposure,
defined, 15
social gatherings, 41–42
swimming, 44

F
face as public symbol, 87
face shields
children, 50
general, 36, 42–43, 49, 60,
97
filter in cloth mask, 31–33,
35, 82
filtration efficacy
fabrics in cloth mask,
70–71
N95 respirators, 72
surgical masks, 72
fit of face mask
beards, 34
mask, 33
flu pandemic of 1918, 87–
88, 88
flu vaccination

general population, 25–26
hospital workers, 25
four-point safety strategy, 12,
    16, 22, 25, 28–29, 41, 50,
    57, 72, 86, 95

G
gaiters, 34–35
Gawande, Atul, 8–9
Germany, 79
glasses, 33, 36, 55
goggles, 36
Goldman Sachs research, 10,
    96
gyms, 40, 43, 74

H
hair salons, 4–6, 42
hand sanitizer, technique,
    17–18
hand washing, 12, 16–18,
    22–24, 33–34, 40–42, 44,
    50–51, 57–58, 61, 72–74,
    86, 89, 95
herd immunity
    concept, 93
    Re, 93–96
history
    1918 Spanish flu, 87–88
    surgical masks, 72
Hong Kong, 14, 72–74
hospital visits, 19, 26, 42

hotels, 42–43
household
    flu shot, 25–26
    infected member, 46
    pets, 49
    quarantine, 47
    quarantine ending, 48
    risk, 47

I
individual blame, 30
influenza *see* flu vaccination

K
KN95 respirators, 37

L
longitudinal studies, clusters
    in community, 73–74, 76

M
mandates by states, 28, 30,
    77–78, 87, 92, 96–99
mask type
    clear mask, 35
    cotton, 32
    double layer, 31
    exhalation valve, 37–38
    fabric, 32–35
    face shield. *see* face shields

filter, 35
gaiter, 34–35
goggles, 36
homemade, 32–33
mask wearing
    medical reasons not to
        wear, 53–54
    prevalence, 10
    put on, 33
    removal, 34
    running, 43–44
    storing, 34
    wash, 34
Mass General Brigham
    (MGB)
    description, 6–7
    flu vaccination program,
        98–99
    research study, 9–11
    safe care commitment,
        24–25
    safety committee, 25, 91
    service center, 26–27
    sick pay, 27
    universal mask policy, 8–9
mathematical modeling
    ABM, 81–83
    R0, 80
    SEIR, 81–82
medical conditions and
    vulnerability, 22, 27, 39,
    41, 64
medical privacy, 30, 63
meta-analysis, 74–76, 92

N
N95 respirator
    description, 37
    exhalation valve, 37
    filtration efficacy, 37
    KN95 respirators, 37
    protection of wearer, 37

O
observational studies
    case clusters in Hong
        Kong, 73–74
    general, 72–73
    hair stylists, 4–6
    households in Beijing, 73
    meta-analysis, 74–76
    MGB, 6–11
    Skagit Valley Chorale, 1–4
occupational health services,
    26, 91
oxygen depletion, 53, 55, 89

P
pets, 49
population-based studies
    German regions, 79
    mathematical modeling,
        80–83
    United States, 77–78
precautionary principle,
    85–86
privacy rights, 30, 63

psychological positive effects, 90

Q

quarantine
  general requirement, 46–47
  household, 47–48

R

R, 80, 93
R0 (R naught), 80, 93
Randomized control trials, 76–77, 83–85
Re
  general, 88
  mathematical modeling, 80
Redfield, Robert, 9–11
remote work, 26, 58–59, 61, 64
restaurants, 5, 13, 20–21, 29, 41, 74
return to work see workplaces, sick pay, 27
running, 40, 43–44

S

school, 1, 49–50, 88
science, its importance, 23, 28, 98

SEIR mathematical modeling, 81–83
self-protective of wearer, 13
sick pay, 27–28
Skagit Valley Chorale, 1, 4, 99
skin problems, 53–54
social distancing
  break rooms, 25
  density rules, 20
  description, 20
  enforcement, 5
social events, 41
social networks, 81, 89
state mandates, studies of mask wearing, 77–78
state re-openings, 4–5, 23, 28–30, 80
superspreader events, 13
surgical masks
  filtration efficacy, 13
  general, 36
  history, 87–88
  polypropylene, 36
Sweden, 93
swimming, 40, 44
symptom check, 12, 16, 18–20, 25

T

testing, 3, 5–6, 8–9, 15–16, 25–28, 44, 56, 62–65, 73, 93

transmission of infection
    children, 49
    droplet transmission, 13,
        67
    without symptoms, 39
transportation, 20–21, 29,
    34, 63, 77, 79

U
universal need for masks,
    6–12, 14–15, 24–30,
    38–39, 42, 48, 50, 58, 61,
    66, 68–69, 73–74, 76–77,
    79–81, 83, 87–88, 90–98

V
vaccination, 10, 25–26, 48,
    59, 93–96, 98

W
washing hands *see* hand
    washing
WHO, 13
workplace safety
    accommodations for
        disability, 61–62
    employee privacy rights,
        63
    employer required, 61
    exposure length, 63
    general, 57–59
    remote work, 64
    return to work, 65
    testing, 62–63
    work-related
        determination, 60